A Primer on Mental Disorders

*A Guide for Educators,
Families, and Students*

Thomas E. Allen, M.D.
Mayer C. Liebman, M.D.
Lee Crandall Park, M.D.
William C. Wimmer, M.D.

The Scarecrow Press, Inc.
Lanham, Maryland, and London
2001

SCARECROW PRESS, INC.

Published in the United States of America
by Scarecrow Press, Inc.
4720 Boston Way, Lanham, Maryland 20706
www.scarecrowpress.com

4 Pleydell Gardens, Folkestone
Kent CT20 2DN, England

British Library Cataloguing-in-Publication Information Available

Library of Congress Cataloging-in-Publication Data
A primer on mental disorders : a guide for educators, families, and students /
    Thomas E. Allen ... [et al.].
       p. cm.
    Includes bibliographical references and index.
    ISBN 0-8108-3919-9 (alk. paper) — ISBN 0-8108-3920-2 (pbk. : alk. paper)
      1. Mental illness. 2. Psychiatry.   I. Allen, Thomas E.
    RC454 .P684 2001
       616.89—dc21   00-067053

The authors dedicate this guide to the countless number of educators, students, and families who have been involved in one way or another with mental illness. It is our hope that this book will aid in the development of educated communities of caring to assist those in need.

The web of our life is of a mingled
yarn, good and ill together.

William Shakespeare, *All's Well That Ends Well*, 1606

Contents

Foreword

It is a pleasure and an honor to have been asked to write the foreword to this book, because I share with the authors the desire to more fully inform our diverse population about mental health and mental disorders—especially those now coming of age. Health care professionals and educators are increasingly aware that good mental health is fundamental to good general health. The recent *Report of the Surgeon General on Mental Health* states that "Tragic and devastating disorders such as schizophrenia, depression and bipolar disorder, Alzheimer's disease, the mental and behavioral disorders suffered by children, and a range of other mental disorders affecting nearly one in five Americans in any year have continued to frequently be spoken of in whispers and shame." Societal prejudices and the stigma about mental illness will only be changed when we each take the time to investigate and educate ourselves and others about normal childhood development and the misunderstandings that deprive our young citizens of appropriate medical care and societal support.

In the 1990s the World Health Organization looked at the various diseases and health conditions that affect the world's population and estimated the global "burden of disease." In the advanced economy of the United States, mental illness was the second major cause of disability and early death. Tragically, almost half of Americans who suffer from a severe mental illness do not seek help for it, although the treatments are proven useful and there is often a choice of effective treatment options available. The end result of neglecting these mental disorders can and will be impaired functioning, pain, loss of freedom, disability, and even death.

Research continues on mental illness as well as all medical illnesses. While much awaits further scientific investigation, some things are now clear. We know that mental health and illness are in a vital changing balance that reflects the sum total of each individual's genetic inheritance and life experience. Throughout a child's development, the brain interacts with and responds to multiple influences. We have also learned that no single gene is responsible for any specific mental disorder or behavior. From research we learn that the cause of mental disorders, in fact, lies in some mix of genes and environment. Learning what causes mental illness is of limited value unless we can provide the treatments necessary to deal with these same illnesses. We are now studying the factors that impede or support access to these treatments. Current systems of care create barriers to treatment, and we also know that stigma, ignorance, and fear about mental illness are major obstacles to gaining better mental healthcare for all citizens, especially our youth.

This clear and important book will help every child, adolescent, and adult learn about these real and treatable illnesses. We have little time to waste. Suicide is the third leading cause of death for youths between fifteen and twenty-four years of age and homicide is the second leading cause. These figures have been steadily increasing for over two decades. One has only to watch the evening news to understand that the tragedy of mental illnesses is going unrecognized and untreated. We must do better for the sake of our children, our families, our teachers, and our friends. We have a duty to be informed and begin the process of leading our children into the sunlight of mental health.

Richard K. Harding, M.D.
President, American Psychiatric Association
2001

Preface

The April 1999 shootings by troubled students at Columbine High School in Colorado and such tragedies in other schools around the country have brought home to the authors the merits of having a text for mental hygiene classes that discusses mental illness. A *Primer on Mental Disorders* defines and describes the many forms of mental illness in a simple but organized way without skirting the standard terms that serve as tools to help readers access more knowledge. We expect this work will be used in middle schools, high schools, and colleges to begin the journey to a greater understanding of this subject—we hope that education about mental health and mental illness will become as widespread as sex education is in primary and secondary schools.

Other audiences for this book are school administrators, teachers, parents and staff, and members of the various organizations mentioned in the text. The information provided can facilitate a better exchange between guidance staff and principals and may help parents to grasp what experts are telling them. Why *should* one learn the proper terms and what they mean? Beyond the fact that knowledge is power, ignorance breeds disrespect, whether it is about sex, an ethnic group, or a mental illness. And that disrespect is dangerous—not only to its victims but also to those who ignorantly use it to exclude and devalue others. But to use the terms intelligently, one must know what they mean.

Acknowledgments

We wish to thank the individuals who contributed to this work:

Eloise Liberty, for her tireless efforts and dedicated production work in collaboration with the authors; *Marilyn Mattsson*, whose extensive editorial background in psychological and psychiatric publications provided expertise above and beyond that of the authors; *Carol Allen*, for untold behind-the-scenes advocacy and support work; *Carolyn Weaver*, for high-quality indexing; *Anne Fredenburg Dolan*, for initial direction on the formatting of content for both educators and the adolescent reader; *Vivia Chang*, for providing insight into the use of the book by school counselors and advisors; *Patricia Ann Martin*, *Ed.D.*, Director, Education for Health and Wellness, Johns Hopkins University, for adding resources pertinent to high school and college students and their families; and *Mary Park*, President, Information Consultancy, Production Editor of this book and author of appendix D, for coordination and support among all of the above mentioned, and for advice and development of valuable content in the area of electronic resources in the appendixes. Mary has been invaluable—her commitment and quiet, gentle, thoughtful manner and wisdom helped solve many knotty problems and made the work more enjoyable than it otherwise would have been. We are very grateful and indebted to her.

Thomas E. Allen
Mayer C. Liebman
Lee Crandall Park
William C. Wimmer

Introduction

Many of the disorders discussed in this book have a long history—some were first described by Greek writers more than two thousand years ago. Systematic disease classification in the modern era can be traced to the end of the nineteenth century, when there was a need to standardize usage across countries and in teaching centers for the purpose of planning, teaching, and research. To start, the First Revision Conference of the International List of Causes of Death (later the *International Classification of Diseases*) was held in Paris in 1900. Then the Committee on Statistics of the "American Medico-Psychological Association" (later the American Psychiatric Association) proposed an early handbook to collect valid data from hospitals for the mentally ill. This handbook was adopted by the association in 1917 and listed a limited number of disorders. World War II showed that the system then in use, mostly for hospital care, was not helpful for 90 percent of the cases handled. For example, it did not identify the more subtle spectrum of disorders that kept young adults from serving in the armed forces but were not severe enough to require hospital treatment. Following some attempts to correct the omission, the American Psychiatric Association finally assembled a distinguished panel of psychiatrists who revised and codified mental disorders in a manual called the *Diagnostic and Statistical Manual of Mental Disorders* (DSM, 1952).

This manual is now in its fourth edition (*DSM–IV–Text Revision*), which was published in 2000. It is used by most American doctors and many others worldwide to classify the diverse forms of mental illness. Rarely do patients have every symptom or sign of an illness, either physical or mental, but there is a threshold that allows the diagnosis to be made by a trained expert. We should remind the reader that these classification schemes do not classify people, but disorders that people may have.

Our book is arranged like *DSM–IV–TR*, using the same "disorder" headings. Our definitions and symptom portraits use reader-friendly language and substitute short words for longer ones, common words for novel ones, and neutral words for words that can be seen as more negative. The *Primer* has been written to be understood by a reader at the tenth-grade level; the style is conversational rather than scientific, and the goal is to be easily mastered rather than rigorous. It is more encouraging than some writing in the field and reflects the authors' combined experience treating patients (see "About the Authors" at the end of the book).

We address most of the major diagnoses, but do not include those we feel are more obscure and rare, so as to make the book more useful and easier to follow for the general reader. We want to provide the best possible sense of the categories and their major features. For the rarer syndromes, the reader is referred to *DSM–IV–TR* itself; however, we think we can orient even those readers. If a reader wants to find a particular syndrome, look in the index; if the numerical code is known, check appendix A which lists all the diagnoses by number.

The "Treatment" part of the format is broken down into "Self-Help" and "Professional Help." Under "Self-Help," the book lists support and self-help groups, survivor accounts, and includes some simple mental hygiene advice. A more complete list of support and self-help groups is in appendix B, along with publisher information for books mentioned in the text. Under "Professional Help" we report the major types of treatment: psychotherapy, medication, and hospitalization. Professional organizations and federal agencies are listed alphabetically in appendix C. Appendix D has additional Web sites for ready classroom access.

We do not discuss any special medications or even classes of drugs because that can become a book in itself and is also soon out of date. We cover neither the variety of psychotherapies that exist nor different hospital programs. Our goal is to be the first resource the public turns to, not the last, and to provide a useful overview of mental disorders.

T. Allen

Chapter 1
Disorders Usually First Diagnosed in Infancy, Childhood, or Adolescence

Section 1: Mental Retardation

Slow and steady wins the race.

> Aesop, "The Hare and the Tortoise," 550 B.C.

What Is the Definition?

Retardation comes from the Latin *retardare*, meaning "to be slow, loiter, or linger"; *mental retardation* is a slowness of mental progress. It is observed in childhood before the age of 18 and can be confirmed by intelligence quotient (IQ) tests that show a mental age significantly below the birth age ("retardation" translates to an IQ of 70 or lower).

What Are the Symptoms?

Mental retardation may be first noticed in infancy or early childhood by a marked delay in reaching the normal milestones of sitting, crawling, walking, and talking. In more subtle cases, it may be observed in school years through the trouble the child has in attaining the skills and concepts that other children are learning at the same age. The youngster's failure to work independently and meet the common demands of his or her age are often what brings the child to the concern of an expert and leads to evaluation.

Subtypes of mental retardation are defined on the basis of IQ scores: mild mental retardation, an IQ of 50–70; moderate, 35–50; severe, 20–35; and profound, below 20. There tends to be a five-point margin of error between one group and the next. Most common are the mildly retarded; the profoundly retarded are the least common.

Who Is Affected?

Retardation is slightly more common among males than females and is present in about 1 percent of the population. For almost half of the affected group, there is no clear cause. For the rest, the types of causes that are known are genetic factors, prenatal factors, delivery problems, infections, trauma, or toxins in childhood.

Onset and Course

The more severe the mental retardation, the sooner it tends to be noticed. Some mildly retarded persons are not identified until their school years, when their deficits disrupt learning tasks, and often later vanish back into the rest of the population as adults.

Although many persons with mental retardation are passive and dependent, some may be aggressive and impulsive. In severe forms, the aggression is turned against the person's own body, for instance, hitting and biting oneself. Other *DSM–IV* disorders that may occur with retardation are: Attention-Deficit/Hyperactivity Disorder, mood disorders, and psychosis. In certain genetic forms, the course and related ailments may be determined by the specific disorder. An example is Down (or Down's) Syndrome, in which congenital heart defects, acute leukemia, and dementia of the Alzheimer's type may occur.

Treatment

Self-Help. National and State Alliances for Retarded Citizens provide advocacy and help to both families and the patient. There are also some disorder-specific groups, for instance, the National Down Syndrome Congress, National Down Syndrome Society, and National Fragile X Foundation (see appendix B). There are some useful books as well, such as *Leslie's Story: A Book about a Girl with Mental Retardation* by Martha McNey and Leslie Fish.

Professional Help. The need for expert help will vary with the degree of impairment. Some children may need formal help only during school years and after that are able to work well and form their own families. Others at the profound level will require residential care all of their lives and may only achieve the most simple level of motor development and self-care. Most of the mentally retarded fall between these two extremes. Urban areas often have a broad array of aid to help families who wish to keep a mentally retarded relative at home. For those who prefer a site away from home, there are supervised community settings, group homes, and residential placements. There are also vocational training programs, sheltered workshops, and programs to help the more severely impaired with motor and self-help skills; clear positive rewards for good conduct often go a long way in shaping behavior. Some individuals may profit from proper psychiatric medication to control impulsive or aggressive behavior.

Classroom Guides. Will vary by the functional level.

T. Allen

Section 2: Learning Disorders

And gladly wolde he lerne, and gladly teche.
                                   Geoffrey Chaucer, *Canterbury Tales*, 1387

What Is the Definition?

Learn comes from the Latin, meaning "track" or "furrow." Learning disorders reflect an impaired ability to track or follow the teaching.

What Are the Symptoms?

Children with learning disorders often have difficulty learning reading or mathematics or demonstrate written expression that is significantly below what would be expected for the child's age, level of schooling, and IQ. Learning disorders are different from learning *difficulties* caused by poor teaching, cultural factors, or lack of opportunity and commonly occur in individuals with disorders of conduct, attention deficit, or depression. Although children without emotional problems may have a learning disorder, low self-esteem and social skill problems may appear secondary to the learning disorder.

Who Is Affected?

Reading disorders are more commonly identified in boys than in girls, perhaps because they come to the teacher's attention due to behavioral problems. Reading disorders occur in 4 percent of school-age children and mathematic disorders in 1 percent. Learning disorders are more common among brothers, sisters, and parents of a child with a learning disorder.

Onset and Course

Learning disorders are noticed after the affected children have started school and failed to achieve. With early help, the children may learn reading, mathematics, and writing adequately for their age and educational level. The disorders, however, may persist into adult life and impair later studies and work.

Treatment

Self-Help. Parents may tutor children. There are also support groups, such as the

Learning Disabilities Association of America, for parents of children with learning difficulties.

Professional Help. Public schools are required by law to develop programs to treat and correct learning disorders.

Classroom Guides. The remediation for learning disorders is primarily educational, although children with low self-esteem or other disorders may require treatment by a mental health expert.

W. Wimmer

Section 3: Motor Skills Disorder— Developmental Coordination Disorder

He that strives to reach the stars often stumbles at a straw.
Edmund Spencer, *The Shepheardes Calendar,* 1579

What Is the Definition?

Coordinate comes from the Latin, meaning "to set in order" or "regulate." With Developmental Coordination Disorder, the child is unable to regulate motor skills.

What Are the Symptoms?

The child may be clumsy and have problems walking, talking, crawling, sitting, buttoning, zipping, and the like at the age these skills ordinarily occur in other children.

Who Is Affected?

Motor Skills Disorder is fairly common and is found in as many as 6 percent of children five to eleven years of age.

Onset and Course

This disorder is first noted when the infant does not roll over or sit at the usual age. It is commonly associated with other delays, such as in developing speech. Some children eventually develop motor proficiency, but for others, coordination problems continue throughout adolescence and adulthood.

Treatment

Self-Help. Parents may help a child practice various motor skills in a patient way. Routine visits to the family doctor will establish the diagnosis.

Professional Help. Occupational therapists or physical therapists may prescribe specific activities that will help the child develop coordination skills.

Classroom Guides. The preschool teacher may bring the child's coordination difficulties to the parents' attention. The teacher may also work with other professionals to help the child improve motor skills.

W. Wimmer

Section 4: Communication Disorders

And Moses said unto the Lord, O my Lord, I am not eloquent, neither heretofore, nor since thou hast spoken unto thy servant: but I am slow of speech, and of a slow tongue. And the Lord said unto him, Who hath made man's mouth? or who maketh the dumb or deaf, or the seeing or the blind? have not I the Lord?

Exodus 4:10–11, the Bible, King James Version

What Is the Definition?

Communicate comes from the Latin, meaning "to pass something along." Communication disorders affect the child's ability to express and receive speech or written language.

What Are the Symptoms?

The child may have a hard time expressing him- or herself, receiving language, or both, as shown on testing. Other children may have a phonological disorder in which a letter may be difficult to say, such as L, and another sound is used instead, such as R. Lisping is common. Some children may stutter. In this case, a word may be said over and over, such as I, I, I. Rate and rhythm of spoken words may be a problem, often with blocking or pauses.

Who Is Affected?

Expressive language disorder occurs in 3 to 7 percent of school-age children and is more common in boys. A combination of expressive and receptive language disorder occurs in 3 percent of school-age children. Phonological disorder is more common in boys and occurs in about 2 percent of first and second graders. Males stutter more than females (3 to 1). Frequently, there is a family history of a communication disorder.

Onset and Course

Expressive or receptive language problems may occur in the course of development or may be acquired from head trauma, disease, or sickness. The development type is usually noticed by three years of age.

About 60 percent of children outgrow the disorder by sixteen years of age. Approximately one-half with the developmental type of expressive language disorder outgrow it, while the other half experience longer-lasting problems. In the acquired type, the course is related to the extent and site of the injury to the brain.

Treatment

Self-Help. Support groups, for instance, TALK (Taking Action against Language Disorders for Kids), may help those who stutter, as well as their families.

Professional Help. Speech therapists are able to offer help. Special education may help those with expressive, receptive, or mixed language problems.

Classroom Guides. Preschool teachers may be the first to identify a communication disorder. Experts in special education are most important in helping these children. Mental health professionals may aid in diagnosis and provide help to the child whose self-esteem suffers as a result of the disorder.

W. Wimmer

Section 5: Pervasive Developmental Disorders

If a man does not keep pace with his companion, perhaps it is because he hears a different drummer.

Henry David Thoreau, *Walden*, 1854

What Is the Definition?

Develop comes from the French *developper*, meaning "to unwrap." With a Pervasive Developmental Disorder, the unfolding bud—the child—is severely affected. The infant's or child's social, psychic, and language growth are very impaired throughout all aspects of the child's development.

What Are the Symptoms?

There are four types of Pervasive Developmental Disorders, defined by age of onset or severity of symptoms: Autism, Rett's Disorder, Childhood Disintegrative Disorder, and Asperger's Disorder. *Autism* is often detected in early infancy. *Rett's Disorder* follows a period of normal functioning after birth and usually appears in the first or second year of life. It is usually associated with severe retardation. The symptoms of Rett's Disorder are similar to those of autism. *Childhood Disintegrative Disorder* follows at least two years of normal development and is often associated with severe retardation. The symptoms are like those of autism. *Asperger's Disorder*, which only involves severe deficits in social interaction, is usually recognized somewhat later than autistic disorder.

With these disorders, the infant or child does not bond, connect, or respond to parents or others in common ways, such as eye contact, smiling, or laughing. Speech and language are impaired or odd. The same words or phrases may be said over and over, although nothing is learned from them. Body movements are awkward or strange and include rocking, dipping, swaying, or clapping. The child may not be aware of others, causing him or her to appear bizarre. Play and games may be rote and rigid. The child may insist on sameness. Moving objects, such as wheels, fans, or doors, may be of great interest. IQ is low in some types.

Who Is Affected?

Males are at much greater risk for Pervasive Developmental Disorders, except for Rett's Disorder, which is seen only in girls. Autism is thought to occur in two to twenty cases per ten thousand individuals and may occur in siblings. The other disorders are more rare. The number of cases of Asperger's Disorder in the population is unknown.

Onset and Course

There are several subtypes of this disorder, some types being more severe than others. Speech, language, and intelligence are not impaired in Asperger's Disorder. Often, but not always in the other disorders, the IQ is low, and seizures and other medical problems may be present.

Symptoms are most often lifelong. In less-severe forms, the person may be able to work, have friends, and take care of him- or herself. Other sufferers may require sheltered living settings.

Treatment

Self-Help. The Autism Society of America provides support, education, and a service index to parents and persons in need. There is also the Online Asperger

Syndrome & Support Group™ (O.A.S.I.S.)Web site. Finally, the movie *Rain Man* (1988), in which Oscar-winning actor Dustin Hoffman portrays an adult with autism, provides insight into the disorder.

Professional Help. The law requires that all children have the right to a free and equal education in the least restrictive environment, and therefore all schools must work with students with special needs and their parents. Schools can provide speech therapy, occupational therapy, and mental health treatment. Doctors are an important part of the child's care.

Classroom Guides. Autistic children require special education from early childhood on. Children with Asperger's Disorder may be taught in a regular classroom, because speech, language, and intelligence are not affected. They may also benefit from social skills groups.

W. Wimmer

Section 6: Attention-Deficit and Disruptive Behavior Disorders

"Reeling and Writhing, of course, to begin with," the Mock Turtle replied, "and the different branches of Arithmetic—Ambition, Distraction, Uglification, and Derision."

Lewis Carroll, *Alice's Adventures in Wonderland*, 1865

Attention-Deficit Disorder (ADD)

What Is the Definition?

Attend comes from the Latin *attendere*, meaning "to apply the mind to." Attention-Deficit Disorder (ADD) thus refers to a child who is easily distracted and unable to apply his or her mind to a given task.

What Are the Symptoms?

Children who suffer from ADD are often messy and careless and do not seem to listen. In school, they may be thought of as class clowns and given the label of "does not play well with others." The children may be bossy and into everything without regard for safety or social norms for their age. They avoid tasks that call for sustained mental effort. They lose toys, school supplies, and track of time. Some children seem driven to flit quickly and without logic from object to object and task to task. They may be loud and chatter all the time. They do not respond well to requests or orders.

Teens and adults with the problem may be less restless but cannot stay focused on a task. Learning is often very impaired. Children with this disorder may be irritable. In children and adolescents, irritability may also be the primary symptom of depression or bipolar disorder; sorting out whether the irritable child or adolescent suffers from ADD, bipolar disorder, or depression is important but sometimes difficult for the mental health professional.

Who Is Affected?

The disorder is much more common in males and is usually present before the age of seven. It affects 3 to 7 percent of school-age children. Fathers and brothers may also have some similar symptoms of ADD.

Onset and Course

Birth trauma, or other damage to the brain, may play a role in the occurrence of ADD in some children, but often such history is not present.

The restless, driven, "hyper" signs of ADD may decrease or not be present when sufferers reach their teen or adult years. Some children eventually make up for their learning problems and do well later in school and at work, but some cases of ADD persist into adulthood.

Treatment

Self-Help. Parents and teachers may help children with ADD by placing them in kind but highly structured settings. Controlled playgroups may help with social skills. Parents and teachers may improve the child's actions by rewards and praise for learning, staying on task, and showing good social skills. There are a number of support groups, including the National Attention Deficit Disorder Association, Children and Adults with Attention-Deficit/Hyperactivity Disorders, Attention Deficit Information Network, and ADD Anonymous.

Professional Help. Prescribed drugs are often useful in helping the child focus and attend, heed requests, and learn in school. Special classes may be in order to help the child gain new ways to learn. Psychotherapy may improve self-esteem and work out other problems causing the restless, driven actions.

Classroom Guides. The diagnosis of ADD is often made by a family physician or mental health expert and teacher working together. Most schools have behavioral checklists designed to rate the child's ability to attend and follow through on tasks. A checklist may also be available through the mental health expert. The same instrument is used at intervals to assess the effectiveness of therapy, medication, and educational interventions.

W. Wimmer

Disruptive Behavior Disorders (Conduct and Oppositional Defiant Disorder)

Snips and snails and puppy dog tails . . .

Robert Southey, *What All the World Is Made Of*, ca. 1862

What Is the Definition?

Disrupt comes from the Latin, meaning "to break apart." Disruptive behavior, then, refers to action by a child or teen that breaks up a social group or home setting, defies a social norm, or shatters the bond with parents and is not useful for group survival or normal for the child's age.

What Are the Symptoms?

Mild forms of disruptive behavior disorders (collectively known as Oppositional Defiant Disorder) may be seen in stubborn, hostile children who refuse to give in to adults or peers, ignore orders, and fail to accept blame for misdeeds. More severe types (Conduct Disorder) are seen in children or teens who bully, are cruel to others, cause fights, force sex upon a victim, set fires, lie to obtain goods or favors, break into property, and defy parental rules. These children show little concern or regard for others.

Who Is Affected?

The disorder occurs more often in urban than in rural settings and usually among children with birth parents who have mood, drug, or Attention-Deficit Disorder problems or who break the law. These children may also have ADD or learning, mood, or drug abuse disorders. Babies who are hard to comfort are more at risk, as are children who have suffered abuse and neglect. Most types of this disorder are more common in boys. Conduct Disorder occurs in up to 10 percent of school-age children.

Onset and Course

Some forms of disruptive behavior disorders begin before age eight, while others start in the teens. The disorder often goes away by adulthood. If there is an early onset, some form may persist and result in antisocial actions and drug abuse in the teens or adult life. Mood and other nervous problems are more common in these children.

Treatment

Self-Help. TOUGHLOVE® groups or parent effectiveness training groups may support parents in gaining control of the child's hostile actions. Special schools or foster homes may assist the child in gaining control of him- or herself. Families-Anonymous World Service Office is a self-help support organization for families of these children.

Professional Help. Parents may need advice from mental health experts. Group treatment is often useful. Drugs prescribed by doctors may assist some children in gaining control of themselves.

Classroom Guides. Incentive programs that reward desired behavior are more effective than those that deprive or punish. Very disruptive children require self-contained classrooms with a high teacher-to-student ratio. Some children with Conduct Disorders may need a residential treatment center.

W. Wimmer

Section 7: Feeding or Eating Disorders of Infancy or Early Childhood

Nebuchadnezzar . . . was driven from men and did eat grass as oxen.
Daniel 4:25, the Bible, King James Version

What Is the Definition?

Eat comes from the Latin, meaning "to be taken in the mouth and swallowed to provide fuel to grow."

What Are the Symptoms?

There are three early childhood eating disorders: *Pica* is a disorder in which the infant eats items with no food value, such as paint, plaster, clay, or feces (*pica* is Latin for "magpie," birds that eat almost anything). *Rumination Disorder* involves the child who eats, then vomits the food, chews it, and swallows it again. The other feeding disorder of infancy or early childhood involves a child who for no known reason does not eat and fails to gain or may lose weight.

Who Is Affected?

Pica is usually seen in mentally retarded infants or children and occurs in 15 percent of adults with severe mental retardation. Rumination Disorder is more commonly seen in infants who have been neglected or abused or have not been stimulated enough. It is rare and is thought to occur more frequently in boys than in girls.

Onset and Course

Feeding disorders in infancy are seen in the first year of life and more commonly in children who have had problem-filled maternal care.

Pica normally lasts for a few months, but may continue into adult life. Medical problems such as lead poisoning, perforation of the bowel, or bowel obstruction may occur. Rumination Disorder often remits spontaneously in infants, but may result in weight loss or failure to thrive. Rarely, it may have a continuous course. Children with feeding disorders in infancy or early childhood often improve and resume growth.

Treatment

Self-Help. Routine visits to the family physician may help prevent feeding disorders. Hot lines and other self-help organizations may help parents avoid abuse of their children.

Professional Help. Mental health interventions oriented toward the parents are essential for problems of neglect, abuse, or lack of stimulation of their child.

W. Wimmer

Section 8: Tic Disorders

One-woman waterfall, she wears
Her slow descent like a long cape
And pausing, on the final stair
Collects her motions into shape.

X. J. Kennedy, *Nude Descending a Staircase*, 1961

What Is the Definition?

Tic comes from the French *tic*, meaning "twitching." Tic Disorder describes a child who has twitches.

What Are the Symptoms?

The symptoms of Tic Disorder occur involuntarily and may include eye-blinking, neck jerking, coughing, sniffing, grunting, barking, touching, stamping, smelling an object, or cursing. A twitch of muscles, often those of the face, that has become a habit may be stopped for varying lengths of time. Included in this category is Tourette's Disorder, which involves more than one motor or vocal tic and results in impaired social or workplace behavior. Obsessions and compulsions may occur with Tourette's. Certain drugs make the tics worse.

Who Is Affected?

Tourette's Disorder is three times more common in boys than in girls. About five to thirty children per ten thousand are affected.

Onset and Course

Tourette's usually begins about age seven but can occur as late as age eighteen. There is a genetic basis for the tics.

Although tics often are lifelong, they may stop for weeks or years, decrease during teen and adult life, or vanish by young adulthood.

Treatment

Self-Help. The Tourette Syndrome Association, can provide peer support and education. A movie called *The Tic Code* (2000, rated R) tells the fictional story of an eleven-year-old with Tourette's examining the shame that patients with this disorder may have.

Professional Help. In diagnosing Tic Disorder, a doctor must make sure that other diseases are not causing the tics. Medications may be recommended by the doctor to help control the symptoms.

Classroom Guides. Children whose symptoms are severe and cannot be controlled by medication require a small, self-contained classroom.

W. Wimmer

Section 9: Elimination Disorders

At first the infant,
Mewling and puking in the nurse's arms.

William Shakespeare, As You Like It, 1598

What Is the Definition?

Eliminate comes from the Latin, meaning "to expel from the body." A child with Elimination Disorder does not have age-appropriate control of bowel and bladder.

What Are the Symptoms?

The child fails to gain control over bowel or bladder by the age of four or five. Some children retain feces, causing a hard stool to form in the bowel. Soiling is due to leaking around the hardened stool. Other children soil with bowel movements normal in shape and form. Voiding of urine in the bed (bed-wetting) or clothes may occur during the day, but most often happens at night. Bowel and bladder training that occurred at a younger age may later break down.

Who Is Affected?

Bowel soiling occurs in 1 percent of five-year-olds. Nighttime bed-wetting occurs in 5 to 10 percent of five-year-olds but decreases to 3 to 5 percent of ten-year-olds, while only 1 percent are symptomatic at age fifteen and older. Boys are at higher risk.

Onset and Course

A physician can determine whether the cause is physical or psychological. Stress, such as divorce, abuse, or birth of a sibling, may cause bowel or bladder training to break down, although some children never obtain total control by the age of four or five. Brothers, sisters, and parents may also have been bed-wetters.

The child often outgrows the problem. Self-esteem, though, may be very impaired by the failure to gain control of body functions. Children often hide soiled clothing and feel ashamed.

Treatment

Self-Help. Parents may help the child gain control by setting times for bowel and bladder release. Rewards for desired habits can be helpful. A bell and pad that sets off an alarm when the child wets at night may help the child learn to wake up in time to avoid a wet bed. Parents may wake the child during the night to go to the bathroom. There is also the National Enuresis Society, from which families can get information and support.

Professional Help. A doctor must make sure the child is healthy and growing well. Sometimes hardened stools must be removed upon the doctor's advice. Parents may need help with child-rearing techniques and learn how to decrease excess stress on the child. The child may need the help of a trained mental health worker to work out the causes of the failure to gain bowel and bladder control. A doctor may prescribe a drug to help stop bed-wetting or soiling.

Classroom Guides. Often the child with an elimination disorder can control him- or herself in the school, and the condition only becomes apparent at home and in other social situations. If it happens in the classroom, the parents and teacher need to work together to minimize blows to the child's self-esteem.

W. Wimmer

Section 10: Other Disorders

Separation Anxiety Disorder

> Parting is all we know of heaven,
> And all we need of hell.
> > Emily Dickinson, *My Life Closed Twice before Its Close*, no. 1732, undated

What Is the Definition?

Separate comes from the Latin, meaning "put apart." Separation anxiety refers to the feeling that comes when the child is apart from his or her mother or significant caregiver.

What Are the Symptoms?

The child with separation anxiety becomes fearful and very homesick, causing him or her to avoid school, camp, or sleeping away from home. Fears may include worries that the parents have died. Nausea, headaches, and belly pains may occur.

The child's sleep is often disturbed, and the child then comes to the parental bed.

Who Is Affected?

In some samples, the disorder occurs just as frequently in males and females; in other samples, it is more common in females. The disorder occurs in 4 percent of children and early adolescents.

Onset and Course

Culture may play a role in the symptoms of Separation Anxiety Disorder. Onset may occur at preschool age or any time before eighteen years. Most often, it occurs before middle school. A move, a death, or an illness may precede the symptoms. Often, the symptoms come and go, but they may persist for years.

Treatment

Self-Help. Parents may help the child adjust to school or other phobic situations by staying with the child and slowly increasing the time apart from the frightened child.

Professional Help. Behavioral techniques may be helpful at the direction of a mental health worker. Prescribed drugs also offer help. Treatment designed to address underlying issues is often useful.

Classroom Guides. Children who refuse to go to school sometimes must be taught at home until their fears of separation are partially resolved. Children may be reintroduced to the school setting gradually and sometimes accompanied by a parent. Little by little, time in school can be increased and time spent by the parent in school decreased.

Selective Mutism

One summer's eve, when the breeze was gone,
And the nightingale was mute.

Thomas Kibble Hervey, *The Devil's Progress,* 1830

What Is the Definition?

Mute comes from the Latin, meaning "to suppress." *Selective mutism* means "to suppress speech by choice."

What Are the Symptoms?

Willful failure to speak at certain required social times, such as at school, with friends, or while at home, are typical. To be classified as selective mutism, the mutism must occur beyond the first month of school and not be due to shyness or lack of knowledge of the language.

Who Is Affected?

Selective mutism is more common in girls than in boys.

Onset and Course

The disorder often occurs before age five and may last several months or, rarely, several years.

Treatment

Professional Help. There is no known self-help treatment for selective mutism. Treatment of child and parents by a mental health expert is required.

Classroom Guides. A close working relationship between teacher and mental health expert is very important. The teacher's descriptions of the child in class and social situations are helpful for the child's therapist. The therapist may provide advice about helping the child in school.

W. Wimmer

Reactive Attachment Disorder of Infancy or Early Childhood

When the bough breaks the cradle will fall,
And down will come baby, cradle and all.

Charles Dupee Blake, 1846–1903

What Is the Definition?

The word *attachment* comes from the Old French word *attacher* meaning "to tie, or fasten." Reactive Attachment Disorder means the infant or young child fails to emotionally connect or fasten to the primary care giver in reaction to the adult's failure to provide "good enough" parenting.

What Are the Symptoms?

The infant or young child may either be withdrawn, overly watchful and inconsolable (Inhibited Type), or overly friendly with strangers (Disinhibited Type). In the latter one observes that "any lap will do."

Who Is Affected?

This disorder is intended to describe only infants and young children who have been subjected to either prolonged hospitalization, institutional care, many changes in primary care givers, or abuse and neglect. Not all children who are exposed to such deviant care develop this disorder. Although the data are limited, the disorder is thought to be rare.

Onset and Course

The disorder is a reaction that begins before the age of five and its course is influenced by whether adequate care givers can be found to whom the child can attach. Even under the best of circumstances a lifelong pattern of superficial relationships may develop.

Treatment

Self-Help. Parents who are lacking in parenting skills can learn from friends or relatives.

Professional Help. Social agencies are crucial in finding and maintaining a suitable caring environment for the child. Parenting groups are useful in developing child rearing skills in parents.

Classroom Guides. Many schools provide social skill groups for children which help the child learn more adaptive ways of relating to others.

W. Wimmer

Chapter 2
Delirium, Dementia, Amnestic, and Other Cognitive Disorders

This group of disorders occurs in people who have had some kind of trauma, substance abuse, or medical illness that has a direct effect on the brain and how it functions.

Section 1: Delirium

> He's a muddled fool, full of lucid intervals.
> Miguel de Cervantes Saavedra, *Don Quixote de la Mancha*, 1605

What Is the Definition?

The word *delirium* comes from the Latin prefix *de-*, which means "away from," and the Latin word *lira*, which means "a line" or "furrow." People who are delirious move away from their usual behaviors and states of being; their actions are strange and their mental states are confused.

What Are the Symptoms?

People who suffer from delirium have a problem focusing their thoughts. They may ask that a question be repeated, or repeat an answer to a question many times. They may have a problem naming a common object, writing a simple sentence, or speaking in a clear, cogent manner. They may wrongly interpret what is seen or heard, such as thinking that flapping window curtains are ghosts or slamming doors are gunshots. In turn, their actions or responses may become extreme and threatening, for example, pulling out intravenous tubing or getting out of a hospital bed when it is unsafe to do so. Likewise, their emotions may become extreme and the person may become either easily upset, angry, and very frightened, or withdrawn, less responsive, and without visible feelings. All of these symptoms may vary and change in degree over time.

Who Is Affected?

Any person who has a general medical illness, or who has taken a prescribed or illegal drug, or who has been exposed to a toxin may develop a delirium. At any one time, 0.4 percent of adults over age eighteen and 1.1 percent of adults over age fifty-five in the general population may have a delirium. For patients ill in the hospital, up to 30 percent at any one time will have a delirium. For older patients, up to 15 percent are delirious on admission to the hospital. Like the elderly, children have a greater chance to develop a delirium at some time.

Onset and Course

The symptoms of delirium may appear over several hours. General medical illnesses and other causative conditions may include poor nutrition or hydration, infection, low blood sugar, liver and kidney disease, a postoperative state, high blood pressure, or a severe blow to the head. Some drugs or substances that may cause delirium are marijuana, cocaine, LSD, PCP, alcohol, barbiturates, and even certain prescribed drugs; these substances may have been either taken for several weeks or more, or withdrawn too quickly. People over sixty-five years of age develop symptoms more easily. Children often develop a delirium from high fevers and certain medicines.

A delirium waxes and wanes over several hours, but it may continue for several weeks as the illness or toxic drug state that causes it improves or worsens. Symptoms of the bizarre behavior and confused mental state become more or less normal over time as the treatment of the illness or of the toxic drug takes effect. Delirium is the sign of a very serious illness that, if untreated, may lead to death.

Treatment

Self-Help. Being aware that an illness may bring delirium might help the patient and family contact a doctor for treatment. Likewise, knowing that a delirium can come from taking certain toxic or prescribed drugs may alert the patient and family to get early treatment.

Professional Help. A doctor, by taking a good medical history, doing a full physical exam, and getting lab tests, should be able to find the cause of the delirium and treat it quickly to avoid a worsening of symptoms, or even death.

Section 2: Dementia

I am a very foolish fond old man,
    Four score and upward, not an hour more or less
And to deal plainly. I fear I am not in my perfect mind.
William Shakespeare, *King Lear*, 1605

What Is the Definition?

The word *dementia* comes from the prefix *de-*, which means "away from," and the Latin word *mens*, which means "mind." Thus, people who are *demented* are away from their own minds or from their normal thinking, or perhaps "out of their mind." In other words, demented people function less well than normal mentally.

What Are the Symptoms?

Persons with dementia have some of the same symptoms as do persons with delirium, and both illnesses may occur at the same time. Demented people have problems with memory, speech, actions, abstract thinking, judgment, balance in walking, and hallucinations. For example, people with dementia may not know such facts as the name of the president of the United States, where they are presently, or what the year, month, and date are, or they may not be able to do simple math. They may do dangerous things, such as walking into moving traffic, or leaving a gas stove on being unaware that it might cause a fire. Over time, these people need more and more help with everyday tasks of daily living.

Who Is Affected?

The cultural background and education of a person affects the chances of becoming demented. Different populations have different rates of infections, diet defects, brain traumas, seizures, brain tumors, and substance abuse that cause some dementias. However, most dementias appear in older people, especially those past age eighty-five.

At age sixty-five, the prevalence of Alzheimer's Dementia is less than 1 percent. By age eighty-five, prevalence has risen to above 10 percent and by age ninety-five, the prevalence is over 35 percent. Dementias do occur in children and adolescents, mostly from medical illnesses, trauma, tumors, or infections.

Onset and Course

The two most common dementias are Alzheimer's Dementia and Vascular Dementia. In Alzheimer's Dementia, the brain actually shrinks. Certain changes in brain cells also occur. When Alzheimer's Dementia occurs frequently in a family, its symptoms often begin before age sixty-five. At least three kinds of genes have been linked to this illness. It occurs more often in women than in men. This dementia may be referred to as *senility*. In Vascular Dementia, blood vessel changes are followed by symptoms of dementia. In contrast to Alzheimer's type, the onset of Vascular Dementia is often abrupt. Vascular Dementias occur less often than the Alzheimer's type. They begin earlier in life and occur more often in men than women.

Some of the other dementias are caused by (1) viruses, for instance, HIV and Creutzfeldt-Jakob; (2) head trauma; (3) gene defects such as Huntington's Disease; or (4) unknown causes—for instance, Parkinsonism and Pick's Disease. Other dementias are caused by physical illnesses, such as high blood pressure, hormone imbalance, vitamin deficiencies, and infections of the brain, kidney, and liver tissues.

Substances that induce dementias are associated with alcohol, inhalants, sleeping pills, and antianxiety drugs. Toxins that cause dementia include lead, mercury, carbon monoxide, certain pesticides, and industry solvents.

Most dementias worsen over time, and very few can be reversed. Some dementias can be kept from getting worse, such as one caused by a physical illness or where a toxic substance has been taken. People eventually die from medical complications.

Treatment

Self-Help. Persons with dementia need help from their family, friends, and health care givers. Family and friends may attend groups led by health care givers or laypersons to learn more about dementia and how better to cope with this illness. These self-help groups also give support to family and friends who live with and care for such patients. One national self-help and information group is the Alzheimer's Disease and Related Disorders Association. One of several books with information about dementia, amnesia, and delirium is *The 36-Hour Day: A Family Guide on Caring for Persons with Alzheimer's Disease, Related Dementia Illnesses, and Memory Loss in Later Life* by Nancy Mace and Peter Rabins.

Professional Help. Doctors will take a history, carry out a physical exam, and do certain lab tests in order to find what is causing the dementia and how best to treat the disorder. Also, certain psychological tests can be administered to help better understand and treat the disorder. Some medicines can slow the downhill process of Alzheimer's and Vascular Dementias. Both psychotherapy and medicines can counter other symptoms of dementia, such as being depressed or being too agitated.

Section 3: Amnestic Disorder

Pass on, let us pass, all in passing,
    and I will look back many times: The sound of hunting horns
when it dies on the wind, is like our memories.
                    Guillaume Apollinaire, *Cors de Chasse* (Hunting Horns), 1913

What Is the Definition?

The word *amnesia* is derived from the Greek *amnesia*, which means "forgetfulness." A person with an amnestic disorder cannot learn and recall certain facts.

What Are the Symptoms?

Persons with this illness have a problem learning new facts or trying to recall data that were once known to them. For example, a man suddenly cannot recall where he is or what the time is, or cannot recognize his spouse or children. In order to fill in the gaps of recent recall problems, the person may make up stories or pretend to know what is going on. Most people with severe amnesia do not know they suffer from such an illness and may become upset when others confront them about it. The effects of the amnesia vary according to the place and degree of damage to the brain. This problem is seen mostly when one tries to recall or memorize facts. Certain details about the distant past may be recalled better and with greater ease than details about more-recent events; but a person's ability to immediately repeat a string of numbers is typically not a problem in amnesia. In contrast, if there are problems with expressing oneself or giving the name of an object, he or she most likely has a dementia rather than an amnesia. Problems with recall are also seen in delirium and dementia; amnestic disorder will be diagnosed only when these two other disorders are not present.

Who Is Affected?

People who have various medical illnesses that are either acute in onset, as in head trauma, or more chronic in nature, as in drug abuse or medicine side effects, can develop amnesias. The age, gender, or family history does not seem important.

Onset and Course

The onset of amnesia may be acute when the cause is head trauma, stroke, or certain kinds of nerve poisons, or it may appear more slowly in cases of long-term drug abuse, chronic nerve poisons, or lack of certain essential vitamins and minerals. The brain damage is more localized and less severe in amnesia than in delirium and dementia. Some amnesias appear and then vanish after a few hours or a few days.

Most symptoms of amnesia are worse shortly after the trauma but lessen over time up to twenty-four months. However, damage to certain brain structure from some blood vessel clots, surgery, and alcohol may cause an amnesia that never improves.

Treatment

Self-Help. A person can learn to avoid those things that brought on the amnesia, such as excessive use of alcohol or drugs or working in places where toxic compounds may be present. Also, patients may learn new ways to store and recall data. Family and friends can attend self-help groups to learn more about the illness and how to cope with the patient's needs. The Self-Help Information Organization and the book mentioned in the previous disorder, Dementia, would also be helpful to family and friends.

Professional Help. Doctors will use the same methods as discussed in Delirium to understand better what may be causing the patient's amnesia and how best to treat it.

They may prescribe certain drugs that can lessen the patient's problems with recall. Specialists may also be able to help patients to cope better with the illness.

Section 4: Postconcussional Disorder

Float like a butterfly, sting like a bee.

> Boxing credo, devised by aide Drew "Bundini" Brown for
> Muhammad Ali, ca. 1962

What Is the Definition?

Postconcussional Disorder (from the Latin words *post*, meaning "after," and *concontere*, meaning "to shake violently") refers to symptoms that appear after someone suffers an injury or trauma to the head (such as a blow or severe shaking) that causes the victim to lose consciousness for a period of approximately five minutes or more. It may also be termed a "closed head injury."

What Are the Symptoms?

Following a concussion, whether severe or mild, a person may suffer aftereffects, which are referred to as *Postconcussional Disorder*. Seizures may occur for up to six months in severe cases. More commonly, the person may not be able to focus attention, concentrate, perform several mental tasks at one time, or learn and recall facts as well as normal. The person may also become tired more quickly, sleep poorly, suffer from headaches, become dizzy, or lose consciousness. Mood changes are also common; the person may get annoyed quickly without being provoked, or become anxious or depressed. In general, this disorder affects the ability to focus at work, at school, and in social settings. Its duration can be as little as a few days or weeks, or up to three or six months.

Who Is Affected?

Athletes in contact sports are more likely to have a concussion than sedentary students, but Postconcussional Disorder is also common after a car or bicycle accident.

Onset and Course

Symptoms of the disorder occur immediately after the head trauma. Many symptoms are worse at first, but gradually lessen and stop. Some symptoms may appear more slowly, but these too will lessen and abate.

Treatment

Medical Alert. It is very important that anyone suffering a head trauma receive immediate emergency medical attention to rule out the possibility of a severe or life-threatening brain injury, for instance, bleeding in the brain or a fractured skull.

Self-Help. Follow the treatment prescribed by a physician. The Brain Injury Association (see appendix B) may be helpful in providing more information for patient, family, and friends of someone with Postconcussional Disorder.

Professional Help. The patient needs to be under the care of a physician. A neurologist or neurosurgeon may need to consulted if symptoms become severe. A consultation with a mental health specialist for behavioral symptoms may be necessary.

Classroom Guides. In the case of a student suffering from Postconcussional Disorder, teachers and administrators need to work with the student's parents and physicians to create a flexible schedule that takes into account the student's need for rest and possible inability to attend school all day, every day. Special provision for home study may be necessary. If minimum-attendance regulations threaten the student's promotion to the next grade, allowances may be needed to permit a student who is capable of making up the work, or who is achieving at grade level, to pass.

M. Liebman

Chapter 3
Substance-Related Disorders

Section 1: Dependence and Abuse

I do not ask, O Lord, that life may be
A pleasant road
I know too well the poison and the sting
Of things too sweet.

Adelaide Anne Procter, *Per Pacem ad Lucem*, 1858–1860

What Is the Definition?

Abuse comes from a Latin word meaning "to use something away from its purpose." *Substance abuse* is the use of a substance for the wrong purpose. *Dependence* is also from the Latin, meaning "to hang from," and *substance dependence* exists when a person "hangs" upon a substance, that is, a pattern of craving exists, or tolerance has been induced, or withdrawal symptoms have occurred.

What Are the Symptoms?

Substance abuse most often comes to the notice of the affected person, his or her family, or workplace when it disrupts a person's life in some way. For instance, "using" harmful substances may lead to a failure to carry out tasks at work, school, or home. It may cause irritability, agitation, euphoria, or withdrawal that bring about conflict with others. It may show up in a failure to use prudent caution while engaging in such activities as driving. Abuse precedes dependency, which includes the symptoms of abuse, along with the blind use of a substance despite:
- a desire to cut down or stop its use
- knowing that the substance is causing physical or mental problems
- concern that it consumes great amounts of time (and money) to obtain
- learning that continued use requires ever larger amounts of the substance to achieve the same effect (tolerance)
- finding that the substance must be taken to avoid symptoms that result if not taken (withdrawal)

The precise pattern relates to the substance abused or upon which there is dependence.

Who Is Affected?

Young people between the ages of eighteen and twenty-four have the highest rates for use of all mind-changing drugs, including alcohol. Dependence can occur at any age, but its most common onset is in the twenties to forties. It is more likely in males than in females. While culture can play a role in some substance use, there appears with alcohol (the best-studied drug) to be a genetic risk factor also. But even where there is a family pattern, milieu and choice play a role. Studies show that one identical twin may be affected and the other not.

Onset and Course

Often abuse of a particular substance evolves into dependence on the same substance. This progression is more likely if there is a high risk for tolerance or withdrawal. The course for substance dependence is often chronic, lasting for years, with worse and better intervals, for instance, periods of heavy substance intake followed by stretches of nonuse. There are some people who make a complete recovery after only one episode.

Substance use can induce other mental disorders. It can also result in much physical harm, depending on the type of substance used, the means of taking it, and judgment and motor impairment under the influence. Substance abuse increases the risk of suicide and in pregnant women drugs may cross to the fetus and cause changes in vital organs and wrenching withdrawal in the newborn. Half of all highway deaths involve either a driver or pedestrian who is intoxicated. Substances may also release hostile trends that lead to criminal acts. Although alcohol abuse in the form of binge drinking has been decreasing among American adults, it has been rising among college students.

Treatment

Self-Help. The best thing one can do to avoid abuse or dependence is not use substances of abuse. The next best thing is not to use a substance for a purpose other than that for which it is prescribed. There is a problem, though, with regard to some drugs that are often prescribed for other reasons, for instance, opiates, sedatives, hypnotics, and anxiolytics. One should be very careful to take these agents only as prescribed and never forget that one *can* get "hooked" on them. They are useful crutches through a time of crisis, but only rarely should such help be required for more than a few months.

The twelve-step program of Alcoholics Anonymous (AA) has been very helpful for persons with alcohol abuse or dependence in controlling their symptoms. AA's success has spawned similar programs for people with other types of substance abuse or dependence, including Narcotics Anonymous (NA), Cocaine Anonymous World Services, Marijuana Anonymous, and others. Where other substance abuse programs do not exist, some people have found it helpful to go to AA meetings to absorb some of the precepts urged there. Also, programs by allied groups such as Al-Anon, Alateen, and Adult Children of Alcoholics have helped families of members afflicted by these disorders to learn about them and how to respond to substance-induced crises in members with the disorder.

Professional Help. Self-help is often not enough to deal with these disorders. Solo or group guidance and teaching about the medical aspects of the syndrome may be needed. Psychotherapy can help patients to perceive the deeper stresses that make them return to the substance abused or depended on. Blood and urine testing may help a patient confront relapse early. Sometimes, medicine that blocks the effect of the substance, or that causes physical illness when the substance is taken, is a useful aid to giving it up; such medication is available for alcohol, nicotine, and opiate dependence but not for marijuana or stimulants. If other mental disorders are present they should be treated, along with any physical problems, to increase the chance of long-term success. During the first year of abstinence, the person is at greatest risk for return to the drug of choice. A hospital stay may be required to get off the drug and, sometimes, to remove the patient from the lure that the drug presents in their usual milieu. Longer-stay residential programs are required for some cases.

Classroom Guides. Substance use can start very early—even in elementary school. As the use increases, school performance may decline. Discussion in classrooms should begin early, and there are outside resources available. *Angela's Ashes* by Frank McCourt is, among other things, an account of a child surviving the severe alcoholism of a parent and the burden it creates for the family. Susan Cheever's memoir, *Note Found in a Bottle: My Life as a Drinker*, describes her own struggles with alcohol. There are also videos that can be rented through the American Psychiatric Association, including *Kids under the Influence*; *Alcohol, Children, and the Family*; *The Haight-Ashbury Cocaine Film: Physiology, Compulsion, and Recovery*; and *AIDS, Addicts, and Recovery*.

Section 2: Intoxication and Toxic Effects

Upon the first goblet he read this inscription, *monkey wine*; upon the second, *lion wine*; upon the third, *sheep wine*; upon the fourth, *swine wine*. These four inscriptions expressed the four descending degrees of drunkenness: the first, that which enlivens; the second, that which irritates; the third, that which stupefies; finally, the last, that which brutalizes.

Victor Hugo, *Les Miserables*, 1862

What Is the Definition?

Toxin comes from a Greek word that means "poison," and *intoxication* means "to be poisoned." Since the term *poisoned* tends to be reserved for someone who becomes extremely ill or dies of a substance, intoxication has the added sense of a state that can be reversed. Some aspect of the state offers something desired, making the person wish to keep doing it. Many of the substances to be discussed can be lethal poisons (irreversible) at large enough doses.

What Are the Symptoms?

For alcohol: relaxed, "high," talky, short attention, impaired judgment, mood changes, slurred speech, poorer fine motor skills, unsteady gait, blackouts, stupor, and coma. The body can process about one drink per hour; amounts in excess of that will lead to greater intoxication and will require more hours to process.

For amphetamines: "high," talky, increased movement, restless, tense, more thin-skinned, angry, poor judgment, impaired social or work function, rapid or slow heart rate, wide pupils, sweating or chills, nausea or vomiting, weight loss, muscle weakness, chest pain, confusion, seizures. The onset occurs within an hour and lasts four to twelve hours.

For ecstasy: (related to amphetamines) "high," talky, "clarity," touchy/feely, increased energy, rapid heart rate, agitation, teeth grinding, nausea, sweating or chills, blurred vision, faintness, dehydration, seizures, cardiovascular collapse, renal failure, coma. The onset is within an hour and the effect lasts three to six hours.

For caffeine: awake, "wired," tremors, restless, nervous, sleepless, bowel or bladder pressure, muscle twitches, rapid or irregular heartbeat, distress in social or work areas. The symptoms may last two to sixteen hours.

For marijuana: "high," easily amused, self-absorbed, impaired fine motor skills, slowed sense of time, fear, poor judgment, impaired memory, redness of the eyes, dry mouth, increased heart rate, and hunger. When smoked, the peak effect occurs within minutes and lasts three to four hours, although it may persist or recur for twelve to twenty-four hours.

For cocaine: "high," aroused, thin-skinned, tense, angry, poor judgment, rambling speech, paranoia, rapid or slow heart rate, wide pupils, sweats or chills, nausea or vomiting, headache, weight loss, muscle weakness, chest pain, ringing in the ears, psychosis, confusion, and seizures. The onset is very rapid if "mainlined" (injected), smoked, or "snorted" (sniffed), and the peak effect can last for one to three hours with some effect to eighteen hours. Binges over a weekend are common among users.

For hallucinogens (LSD): vivid sensations, fear, depressed mood, paranoia, feeling people are talking about you, fear of losing one's mind, impaired judgment, hallucinations, feeling that things aren't real, wide pupils, rapid heart rate, sweating, heart pounding, blurred vision, tremors, and poor fine motor skills. The hallucinations, as "flashbacks," may recur without use of further hallucinogen. Peak effects may occur within minutes to hours and last hours to days after the dose.

For inhalants (glue, gasoline): "high," hostile, poor judgment, dizzy, impaired fine motor skills, slurred speech, rhythmic eye movements, unsteady gait, slowed down, sleepy, self-absorbed, muscle weakness, blurred vision or seeing double, confusion, and stupor or coma. Peak effect occurs within a few minutes, and may last one to two hours.

For opioids (heroin): "high" followed by distant, slowed, sleepy, self-absorbed state, poor judgment, small pupils, dry mouth and nose membranes, slow gastrointestinal tract, drowsy, slurred speech, slowed breathing, and coma. The degree to which a person is affected depends on the dose and the individual's built-up tolerance; the time span for the symptoms is four to eight hours. If "mainlined" or "snorted," the peak effect occurs within minutes.

For PCP: "charged," talky, hostile, violent, fearful, impulsive, erratic, poor judgment, slurred speech, dizzy, rhythmic eye movements, nausea, increased saliva, rapid heartbeat, higher threshold to pain, staggering gait, rigid muscles, very acute hearing, hallucinations, and seizures or coma. The degree to which a person is affected is linked to the dose. PCP's peak effects occur two hours after oral doses or at once if injected. Effects may last from eight hours to two or three days.

For sedatives, hypnotics, anxiolytics (seconal, halcion, valium): relaxed, "high," mood swings, poor judgment, slurred speech, unsteady gait, rhythmic eye movements, poor fine motor skills, blackouts, stupor, and coma. The peak effect may occur within minutes to hours and the effects may last hours to days.

Who Is Affected?

Anyone who takes enough of any of these substances will show the effects of intoxication.

Onset and Course

Intoxication is sought for its *desired* effects, and the other mental and physical effects are judged as the price that must be paid. The desired effects are what lead to abuse and dependency. The substance meets some felt need so well that seeking it becomes in essence a full-time job. Although inhalants tend to be one of the first substances abused, because of their access (even for young children) through such readily found substances as gasoline or glue, the age of first use of alcohol and many other drugs has dropped over the years and is being seen in younger and younger children. The factors outlined for abuse and dependency apply here.

The intoxication symptoms that are produced by a substance relate to the substance used, its dose, the pattern of use, and traits of the user. For many of these substances, there is risk of death from overdosage. There is also a risk of harm to others, either in drunken rages or by error due to the impaired abilities when the person is driving or using heavy machines. Intoxication can sometimes lead to other mental states that may need acute care. Some people do "age out" of substance use in midlife.

Treatment

Medical Alert. An overdose is a medical emergency, and death can occur.

Self-Help. Because intoxication often leads to repeat use, abuse, and dependency, the self-help treatments are the same as those covered under the self-help heading for "Dependence and Abuse."

Professional Help. The potential for substance abuse and dependency, as well as the acute medical problems resulting from intoxication, warrant medical treatment. It may be necessary to medically manage the more severe effects of these intoxications. There are also some medications that can be used to rapidly block the effects of some drugs—for instance, heroin by naloxone—in cases of overdose.

Classroom Guides. Students who are intoxicated in the classroom will show poor judgment and impaired recall during discussions. If the use is at home during study hours, it may impair the ability to learn new material.

Section 3: Withdrawal

A Hard Rain's A-Gonna Fall

Bob Dylan, song title, 1963

What Is the Definition?

Withdrawal occurs when a person stops ingesting a chemical substance, such as alcohol or nicotine, to which the body has become accustomed and to which it has developed a tolerance. *Tolerance* comes from the Latin word meaning "to bear or endure." In medical terms it means bearing or enduring the substance by fitting one's body to it. Someone who has become *tolerant* to a drug receives less effect at the same dose of the drug and must increase the dose to get the former effect. *Withdrawal* comes from a Middle English word meaning "to take back," and here it means to take back (the self) by giving up the drug or substance. Someone who is a constant user of a substance and has built up a tolerance to it will go through withdrawal symptoms.

What Are the Symptoms?

As a rule, the symptoms of withdrawal are the reverse of those of intoxication. Thus if someone taking a substance enjoyed a "high," they are likely to pass through a "low" when they withdraw. If they felt relaxed, they are likely to feel more tense or edgy; if "aroused," then more slowed or tired. If the person was "talky," he or she may be subdued or suppressed. If the pupils were small, they may be larger than normal during withdrawal; if hunger was suppressed, the desire for food will increase. There are a few withdrawal syndromes that include more than the reverse of the intoxication effects that we shall describe.

Alcohol withdrawal may be marked by sweating, a rapid pulse, restlessness, insomnia, nausea, vomiting, hand tremors, hallucinations, delirium, and even seizures. These symptoms peak by the second day of abstinence and are much better by the fifth day. Some symptoms, though, may continue at low levels for three to six months.

Nicotine withdrawal is announced by craving, tension, depressed mood, being grouchy, scattered thinking, being restless, being sleepless, gaining weight. The symptoms may begin within a few hours of ending smoking and peak in one to four days, but may last for three to four weeks. Low-level symptoms may persist for six months.

Ecstasy withdrawal may be accompanied by depression, sleep disturbance, word-finding problems, and impairment of short-term memory. Psychotic events may also occur weeks or months later.

Opioid (e.g., morphine, heroin, codeine, methadone, Demerol, fentanyl) withdrawal may be attended by craving, being restless, unease, "achy feeling" in back and legs, increased feelings of pain, nausea, vomiting, diarrhea, runny nose, teary eyes, sweating, pupils wider, yawning, fever, insomnia. These symptoms can begin within six to twenty-four hours of the last dose of heroin, peak in one to three days, and subside over five to seven days. This pattern varies with each class of drug in this group.

Sedative, hypnotic, or anxiolytic (barbiturates, such as Seconal; benzodiazepines, such as Xanax, Valium, and Ativan; carbamates, such as meprobamate; and methaqualone, also known as Quaalude) withdrawal is like alcohol withdrawal, even to a risk of hallucinations. There is the greatest risk of seizures in this class of drugs. The onset, time of peak symptoms, and length of total course vary and depend upon the drug that has been used.

Many drugs in the last two classes (*opioids* and *sedative/hypnotic/anxiolytic*) are usually prescription medications, but they are also sold "on the street" illegally under a variety of names. The severity of the syndrome will depend on the drug, the length of time used, and the dosage used.

Who Is Affected?

After frequent use of a substance that can produce tolerance, stopping its use quickly for any reason, whether by choice or because it is not at hand, will produce withdrawal.

Onset and Course

The onset and course of withdrawal have been described above. There are real safety risks to a person withdrawing from drugs in a slapdash manner. In addition to the unpleasant symptoms already mentioned, others include heart attack, seizures, delirium, stroke, or falls.

Treatment

Self-Help. Not getting "hooked," which often means not starting to use these substances, is the best self-treatment. If a doctor has prescribed them for a good medical reason, both patient and doctor must bear in mind the addictive potential and use the drugs only for as long as is absolutely necessary and then taper them down when stopping their use. If tolerance has occurred, and withdrawal is required, medical help really should be sought. Caffeine and nicotine may be the only exceptions, and here, smoking cessation programs can be helpful. If one does not have or does not wish to use a family doctor, the National Drug and Alcohol Abuse Information and Treatment Referral Hotline/National Institute on Drug Abuse Helpline (see appendix C) can provide a referral.

Professional Help. Although it may sometimes be possible to withdraw from the use of alcohol, opiates, sedatives, hypnotics, or anxiolytics outside of a hospital, it often is not. In most cases, a physician's guidance is wise. Alcohol and opiate dependency frequently have other health problems tied to them. Medical help can make the withdrawal safer and less painful.

Classroom Guide. Withdrawal usually requires medical help.

Section 4: Substance-Induced Disorders

How doth the little crocodile
Improve his shining tail,
And pour the waters of the Nile
On every golden scale!

How cheerfully he seems to grin,
How neatly spreads his claws,
And welcomes little fishes in
With gently smiling jaws!

Lewis Carroll, *Alice's Adventures in Wonderland*, 1865

What Is the Definition?

Induced comes from the Latin, meaning "to lead or bring into." Substance-induced disorders are those in which a substance "brings" the user into other mental disorders. And, like the boatman that ferried souls across the River Styx in Greek myths, they do not always bring them back.

What Are the Symptoms?

The symptoms of a substance-induced mental disorder are the same as those of the disorder when not induced by a substance and are described in other chapters, for instance, Delirium, Dementia, Amnestic Disorder, Psychotic Disorder, Mood Disorder, Anxiety Disorder, Sleep Disorder, and Sexual Dysfunction. There is a unique symptom for hallucinogens, known as "flashbacks" or "Persisting Perception Disorder."

Who Is Affected?

Anyone taking drugs is at risk for other disorders that may be induced by those drugs. Anyone with a family history of a major psychiatric disorder should be especially wary.

Onset and Course

Certain types of induced mental illness are more often related to certain substances than to others, and a person's prior response to the substance is a guide to its future effects. The induced ailment may occur in the course of intoxication or withdrawal from the substance and then fade after that state passes, or the symptoms may persist, and even be lasting. The time between the substance use and the onset of a mental illness is a guide to whether the illness has been induced by the substance. A mental disorder that persists more than four weeks after the end of an intoxication or withdrawal is unlikely to be substance-induced, although substance-induced disorders that may persist include dementia, amnesia, and flashbacks.

The induced mental illness may increase the patient's risk of suicide or harm to others. Aside from its effect on the brain, the substance may have a damaging effect on other organ systems (liver, heart, kidneys, immune system, bone marrow, GI tract, pancreas, blood pressure, and reproductive function), as well as the unwished-for side effects of sharing needles (e.g., AIDS, hepatitis, abscesses), smoking (bronchitis, emphysema, cancer), or "snorting" (loss of nasal septum).

Treatment

Self-Help. The best thing that one can do to prevent getting substance-induced disorders is not to use the substance.

Professional Help. Because of the increased risk, these patients should be seen by a professional expert in the field who can make a judgment as to when and how much to treat the induced illness, since it may abate as the patient withdraws from the substance. The approach to the various induced illnesses can be found in the relevant sections of this volume

I. Allen

Chapter 4
Schizophrenia and Other Psychotic Disorders

Long is the way
And hard, that out of hell leads up to light.

John Milton, *Paradise Lost*, 1667

What Is the Definition?

Schizophrenia comes from the Greek *schizo*, meaning "fractured or separated" (hence broken), and *phrenia*, or "mind," thus meaning "broken mind." It is the most common form of psychosis. Psychosis is the loss of the skill to judge what is real in one's contact with the physical and social world. Such people may hear people speaking to them when there is no one there, imagine slights when none were intended, or feel they are singled out for harm by groups or organizations who may even be trying to help them. The person is often in a very fear-filled state.

What Are the Symptoms?

People who suffer from schizophrenia may hear voices, have paranoid ideas, reveal strange thoughts, display odd behavior, be worried and in turmoil, or be very withdrawn. The voices tend to be harsh, condemning, or belittling; they may suggest suicide or self-harming acts or even actions harming someone else. The people may have delusions that they are despised, or feel they are being pursued by someone; they may believe that the radio or TV is speaking just to them and sending them a special message, or that their suffering is a sign of special status, for instance, that they are Jesus or the Antichrist. They may dress in a strange fashion, for example, wearing several layers of heavy clothes even in the summer, and may not bathe, shave, or comb their hair. They may be quite hostile or withdrawn. Modern writers tend to speak of positive symptoms (e.g., hearing voices, delusions, strange behavior) and negative symptoms (e.g., withdrawal, apathy, joylessness). These symptoms sometimes cause family, teachers, or coworkers to suspect they are taking drugs, but a psychiatric evaluation can sort out the true state of affairs.

There are a number of subtypes of schizophrenia based on the foremost set of symptoms, for instance: Paranoid, Disorganized, Catatonic (rigid stupor or very excited), or Undifferentiated. Another subtype, Schizoaffective Disorder, stresses a strong mood aspect as in "high" and "low" moods. The next episode of psychosis may be different from the ones preceding it. There are some subtypes based on the history and course, for instance, Brief Psychotic Disorder (lasting less than a month), Schizophreniform Disorder (lasting one to six months), and Residual Type. There are also psychotic disorders due to physical illness (e.g., brain tumors, infections, endocrine problems) and ones that may be substance-induced. These subtypes cover the main groups in this section; there are others that are very rare and not discussed here.

Who Is Affected?

Although schizophrenia appears in all cultures and epochs, it is less common than mood or anxiety disorders. It occurs in between 1 and 2 percent of the population at large, but if both parents have the disorder, the risk rises to 40 percent, and in identical twins, if one twin has the disorder, the risk rises to almost 50 percent for the other suggesting genetic links (however, with identical genetic endowment in twins, the figure of 50 percent suggests other factors also play an important role). Stress often plays a triggering role, but this is better seen in hindsight.

Onset and Course

The first psychotic break usually occurs between the mid-teens and mid-thirties, but it has been known to occur in children under ten and adults over forty-five. Schizophrenia occurs about equally among males and females; the onset tends to be earlier in males, later in females. It often requires hospitalization, especially for males, and the acute turmoil of the illness may recur. Because of the effort needed to suppress the message of the voices and to try to hide some of the thoughts that the lucid self knows are insane, other functions of the mind are robbed and there may be a decline in school, work, and social performance. Medication can be essential, but there are examples of patients who go on to a successful life without requiring medication. Suicide is a greater danger for this disorder than for any other mental illness besides major depression. The majority of people with Schizophrenia do not marry.

Treatment

Self-Help. There are two self-help groups that can be useful to those suffering from Schizophrenia: "On Our Own" and Schizophrenics Anonymous. In addition, families may find information and support through the Alliance for the Mentally Ill and the Mental Health Association (see appendix B for information). Persons with the disorder need much support, as do their families. After the acute episode resolves, recovery can be facilitated by social integration, but respecting a patient's limits is also important and there may be need for "time outs" during which a patient can withdraw. There are many books about psychotropic medications available that can enable patients and families to get a practical understanding of particular drugs and the newer ones coming on the market.

There are some memoirs about this disorder written by patients and family members which give the reader a firsthand account and feel of what it is like to have the disorder or to have a close family member with it. Some examples include *I Never Promised You a Rose Garden* by Joanne Greenberg, *When the Music's Over: My Journey into Schizophrenia* by Ross Burke, and *My Mother's Keeper: A Daughter's Memoir of Growing Up in the Shadow of Schizophrenia* by Tara Elgin Holley and Joe Holley.

Professional Help. The elements of professional help for schizophrenia include psychotherapy, medication, and partial or full hospital care. They may be used in various combinations as is most fitting for the patient at any given time.

Psychotherapy involves a person talking with a trained professional about his or her life, someone outside the patient's world who can be trusted because they are not involved in the patient's previous struggles and can help the patient look at what happened and what to expect. It may help the patient to learn what stresses to avoid and which to face.

Medication can be essential in easing the acute turmoil and fear, quelling the symptoms, and supporting the will to recover. It is not without its risks, though, including: allergies, drug interactions, risks to the fetus in pregnancy, and side effects and adverse reactions, some of which may be lasting and can be disabling. Talk to a doctor about them. One may wish to consult published books on health for the layperson, or the most current version of the *Physicians Desk Reference*. Many people with this disorder will require some medication for the rest of their lives to keep their symptoms under control, just as patients with severe asthma or severe arthritis do. A minority are able to make a full recovery and do not need it.

Hospitalization may be needed from time to time, when acute breaks occur, to protect the patient or someone else from harm. Sometimes this may be against the person's wishes, but mostly it can be done with his or her accord. The patient may ask for hospitalization, or at least accept it if it is offered, because the person often has some insight into his or her state at the time. A day program may take the place of twenty-four-hour care or permit quicker discharge. At times, a community living unit with other people also on their way back from a severe mental illness may be very helpful. Some expert help should be there for the family as well, to inform them as to the nature and course of the disorder, assist them with crises, and help them put the patient's behavior in a context.

Classroom Guide. Teachers discussing this subject with students may wish to use some of the videos that are available from the American Psychiatric Association, such as *Mental Illness in the Family*, *Recovering from Mental Illness*, *My Sister Is Mentally Ill*, and *Out of My Mind*, which are intimate portraits of psychosis and schizophrenia.

If a teacher suspects a student may be suffering from this disorder, referral for an evaluation by a specialist is crucial and may be life-saving. The teacher's concern should be discussed with both the student and the parent. If a student is known to have this disorder and is in treatment, special handling may be required. A decision may need to be made about special schooling or special provisions in a regular classroom.

T. Allen

Chapter 5
Mood Disorders

Mood is a state of mind or feeling or spirit. The word *mood* comes from the Old English *mod*, which means "disposition." Moods can range from very low, or "depressed," to very high, or "manic." It is normal to have mild mood changes from normal to low when stressed and to joyful when something really good happens. Most people have had times of very low moods, but very high moods are much less frequent.

The two types of mood disorders are Depressive Disorders, in which the only mood problem is depression, and Bipolar Disorders, in which there are manic moods with or without a history of depressed moods.

Section 1: Depressive Disorders

The melancholy days are come, the saddest of the
  year,
Of wailing winds, and naked woods, and
   meadows brown and sere.

       William Cullen Bryant, *The Death of the Flowers*, 1832

What Is the Definition?

The word *depress* comes from the Middle English word *depressen*, which means "to push down." To *be depressed* means to have a "pressing down" of the spirits or to feel "low." A depressive disorder occurs when symptoms cause major distress or trouble in social situations, working, school, or other crucial aspects of daily living.

What Are the Symptoms?

Depressed persons have a depressed mood most of the time on almost every day. Adults by and large know when they are depressed and can describe feelings of painful distress, but children and teens may only know they are angry or cranky or they may "misbehave." Depressed persons have lost the ability to enjoy things or to be interested in doing anything, and they often have weight loss and seriously interrupted sleep (although for some people there may be weight gain or increased sleeping). They may feel very wound up and yet find it hard to be at all active. They often feel very tired and lack vigor. They can feel worthless, with extreme, undue guilt. They frequently have lowered power to think or concentrate and have trouble making up their minds. They can feel hopeless, and they often have thoughts of wishing for death, or suicidal thoughts and plans.

The two major depressive disorders are Major Depressive Disorder and Dysthymic (from the Greek for "bad mind or soul") Disorder. In Major Depressive Disorder, the symptoms cited above are severe, whereas in Dysthymic Disorder, the symptoms are less severe but much more chronic, having been present for at least two years, often since the early teens or even childhood. A Major Depressive Disorder evolves over days to weeks. Anxiety symptoms may have been present for weeks or months prior to the depressed symptoms and may have concealed them for a time.

There are other types of depression, such as those that occur in certain seasons, during major holidays, after childbirth (postnatal), or on a regular basis during the menstrual cycle. In older persons, it can be hard to tell whether symptoms are due to a mood disorder or to a dementia, such as Alzheimer's Disease. In both cases, there can be a depressed mood and a loss of interests, with weight and sleep changes, mental turmoil, and poor ability to think and make up one's mind. Careful evaluation is the key, since in dementia there is a disease that is likely to become worse, and in the other case, there is a mood disorder that can be treated with success.

Who Is Affected?

A nationwide survey found that almost one person in ten had a Depressive Disorder at some point in 1990. Major Depressions occur twice as often in women as in men, while Dysthymia occurs up to three times as often in women, except in childhood where it occurs about equally.

Causes of depression can be roughly listed as "constitutional" or "environmental." With the former, there is often a family history of mood problems. Such families may include people with a high sensitivity to the feelings and needs of others as well as family beliefs and attitudes that foster depression. Environmental causes are countless, including early childhood loss of a parent, child abuse, medical illness, and the many traumas that can occur in one's private and working life.

Onset and Course

Depressions can occur at any age, including early childhood. If not treated, a Major Depression will often last six months or longer. Most people recover fully; however, 40 percent continue to have significant symptoms of the Major Depression for a year or more. A large number of people who have fully or partly improved have one or more later episodes. About 10 percent of teenagers who have repeated Major Depressions later develop Bipolar Disorder.

Depression can threaten life. The most serious possibility is suicide, and this must always be kept in mind in dealing with a person who is depressed. Any sign that he or she might be thinking of suicide must be taken seriously, even if at the moment the person is not planning suicide or seems to be only making a threat or trying to attract attention.

Treatment

Self-Help. People who know that they are depressed can learn ways to help themselves, such as confiding in trusted friends and spouses, engaging in hobbies, and exercising regularly. The more depressed a person is, the simpler such plans usually have to be. There are certain groups that can be helpful, such as the Depression and Related Affective Disorders Association (DRADA), National Alliance for the Mentally Ill (NAMI), and Mental Health Association. There are a number of good books describing personal experiences with depression, including Meri Nana-Ama Danquah's *Willow Weep for Me: A Black Woman's Journal through Depression*, and William Styron's *Darkness Visible: A Memoir of Madness*.

Professional Help. The type of treatment depends on the degree of the depression. In milder cases, talking with one's physician or psychotherapist can help greatly. Often, talking about the symptoms, knowing their cause, and learning that one will most likely recover fully helps the person to find strength to struggle against self-critical ideas and to solve the real-life problems facing him or her. In more severe depressions, psychotherapy with an expert is required, and antidepressant drugs may also be essential. In the case of very severe depression, with or without the risk of suicide, a brief time in a hospital may be required, and in a very small number of such cases, when severe symptoms and the danger of suicide persist, the doctors may suggest a brief course of electroconvulsive treatment.

If depressions recur, "maintenance" drug treatment on a long-term basis may be needed, along with psychotherapy that may be less frequent (e.g., monthly) depending on the kinds of life problems that the person must resolve, including the presence of other psychiatric or medical problems.

Section 2: Bipolar Disorders

Misled by fancy's meteor ray,
    By passion driven;
But yet the light that led astray
    Was light from heaven.

Robert Burns, *The Vision*, 1786

What Is the Definition?

The prefix *bi* comes from the Latin *bis* or *bi*, meaning "two," and *polar* comes from the Latin *palus*, meaning "stake" or "pole." *Bipolar* means having two poles or extremes of moods. A person with this illness must have had at least one "high" or manic phase. These manic states tend to occur in cycles that often—but not always—alternate with periods of depressed moods.

What Are the Symptoms?

The person with a "high," or manic mood is most often very cheerful, which may cause others to feel the same way. The mood is likely to be expansive, in that the person is fervent about many topics and may start talking intimately with strangers. Less often, the major mood is irritable, and the person may become quite angry when there is any dissent or hindrance to his or her wishes. Irritability may be the key symptom in children. Other symptoms and behaviors can include very high trust and belief in oneself despite extremely poor judgment, intense activity with little need for sleep, being in turmoil, and talking nonstop, sometimes with dramatic gestures and sing-song speech. The person may act on impulse with probable distressing results, such as going on buying sprees, engaging in rash sexual acts, or entering into foolish business ventures. In very severe cases, there may be short-lived delusions or hallucinations.

There are three major types of Bipolar Disorder: Bipolar I Disorder, Bipolar II Disorder, and Cyclothymic Disorder. In Bipolar I Disorder, both the manic and depressed states are severe. In Bipolar II Disorder, severe depressed states alternate with milder highs called "hypomanic" moods. Hypomanic moods never include delusions or hallucinations and do not require hospitalization. People with this disorder may even function much better in some ways during these times and may be very successful in careers as a result. However, they can also make the same kinds of errors in judgment as those with true manic states. The hypomanic state, while often sensed by those who are close, may not be seen at all by friends, strangers, or by the affected person. In Cyclothymic Disorder, there are cycles of mild lows and mild highs that have been present for at least two years, of such a frequency that the person has not been without symptoms for more than two months at any one time.

Who Is Affected?

Whereas most people feel depressed at times and significant clinical depression occurs during the lifetime of about one in five people, Bipolar Disorder is much less frequent. There are often relatives with mood disorders, and in the case of identical twins, there is a particularly high chance (75 percent) that if one twin has Bipolar Disorder, the other will have it also. It is therefore thought that Bipolar Disorder has a strong genetic basis, but it is not clear yet whether the basis is for bipolar illness itself or for a poorly regulated response of mood to chronic childhood stresses, such as family conflict and loss. In some cases, mood swings are more frequent in certain seasons. Bipolar Disorder occurs in about equal numbers in males and females.

Onset and Course

A first mood cycle may occur at any age from childhood to old age. Most people with Bipolar Disorder recover fully between periods of illness, but about one in four have continuing signs of mood and work difficulties between episodes. There is an increased frequency of alcohol and drug abuse problems. Rash acts during manic moods can have devastating consequences, such as financial ruin, divorce, and serious legal problems, any of which may be followed by severe guilt-ridden depression and suicide. The course of the disorder can be greatly affected by the person's ability and inclination to see that this is an illness and that he or she must seek help when moods start to change. If the person accepts this, then the illness can be managed with good success. There are a small number of cases in which the mood swings occur more and more often, called "rapid cycling." Three out of four such patients are women. More frequent hospitalizations and very close guidance are required in these cases.

Treatment

Self-Help. A person with Bipolar Disorder may go through a number of manic states before he or she agrees that this is an illness. This is because the manic state feels great, and the person is certain that he or she is in perfect mental health. Local chapters of DRADA, NAMI, and the Mental Health Association can be very helpful. In *An Unquiet Mind* (Vintage Books, 1996), Kay Redfield Jamison, professor of psychiatry at Johns Hopkins University, writes movingly about Bipolar Disorder both from her own personal experience as well as from a professional perspective.

Professional Help. Both medication and psychotherapy are required, and there may be short hospitalizations. There are now a number of drugs for manic states (some of these drugs, known as "mood stabilizers," can also be used to treat epileptic seizures). Most patients must remain on these drugs for a long time and may also need to take antidepressant drugs. When people are getting over manic states, the doctor must be alert to the possibility of sudden swings into depressed states, because a person may now have great shame and guilt after seeing how foolish and even harmful his or her actions were when in the manic state.

L. Park

Chapter 6
Anxiety Disorders

Anxiety Disorders are a group of syndromes in which a heightened state of unease, worry, or fear is the basis for the symptoms. These syndromes are set apart from each other by kinds and degrees of anxious symptoms, along with the ways the individual has learned to try to prevent the symptoms. People with anxiety disorders often have some symptoms of depression and vice versa, and sometimes a person has one or more Anxiety Disorders along with a Depressive Disorder.

The major Anxiety Disorders are Panic Disorder, Phobias, Obsessive-Compulsive Disorder, Posttraumatic Stress Disorder, and Generalized Anxiety Disorder.

Section 1: Panic Disorder and Phobias

The thing I fear most is fear.

Michel Eyquem de Montaigne, *Essays*, 1580

What Is the Definition?

Panic states and phobias are both described in this section. They often occur together in the same person because phobias can arise as ways to try to avoid panic attacks. The word *panic* comes from Pan, a Greek god who was a source of fright or terror to flocks and herds. To feel panic is to be seized by a sudden, frantic feeling of fright and an urgent wish to flee. The word *phobia* comes from the Greek, meaning "fear." People have a phobia when there is an anticipated fear of another person, object, or setting to such a degree that they feel compelled to avoid contact. Very often this contact avoidance occurs following an episode of sudden, extreme, and frantic fear, that is, a panic attack.

What Are the Symptoms?

A Panic Disorder is diagnosed when a person has attacks of panic that occur without warning. These attacks begin suddenly and build up to a peak, usually in less than ten minutes, and are often accompanied by a sense of great danger or doom and an intense urge to escape. Some of the physical and mental symptoms are a rapid and pounding heartbeat, pain or pressure in the chest, feeling short of breath or about to choke or smother, sweating, trembling, nausea, feeling dizzy or faint, feeling unreal, fear of losing control or going crazy, fear of dying, numbing or tingling feelings, and cold or hot sensations. Panic attacks can occur with other anxiety disorders, and the key to diagnosing a separate Panic Disorder is if the attacks occur with no warning.

Just one or two panic attacks can change a person's life, because he or she will likely begin to make urgent efforts to prevent any more attacks. Since the attacks tend to occur without any known rhyme or reason, the person often assumes they can be prevented by staying away from the kind of place where an attack has occurred or where one can imagine it might occur. In this way the person may also develop a certain kind of phobia called Agoraphobia, which refers to the fear of being in places or settings from which it might be hard or awkward to escape, or in which help will likely not come if panic symptoms occur (*agora* is Greek for "marketplace"). This kind of fear tends to expand to the point that eventually the person cannot go to stores, travel, be in a crowd, or in some cases even leave the home. Sometimes a person has only one or a few panic attacks before he or she becomes imprisoned by a highly restrained life, even if the feared panic attacks never or rarely occur again.

There are two other types of phobias that may or may not involve panic symptoms: Specific Phobia and Social Phobia. A Specific Phobia is a marked and lasting fear of certain objects or settings, such as types of insects or animals, heights, bridges, tunnels, flying, elevators, or blood (for School Phobia in children, see chapter 1, section 10, "Separation Anxiety Disorder"). Persons with Social Phobia, which can also be called Social Anxiety Disorder, have a marked and lasting fear of social or performance situations in which they could feel shamed or where others might judge them to be fearful, ineffective, weak, crazy, or stupid. In these types of phobias, any panic symptoms occur in the known feared situations and do not occur out of the blue.

Who Is Affected?

A nationwide survey found that more than one person in ten suffered an Anxiety Disorder. These syndromes are more frequent in women than men, except for Social Phobia where the occurrence is about equal for males and females. All of the Anxiety Disorders result from complex groupings of temperament, environment, and life events. Careful study of a each person's history almost always reveals problems with self-esteem as well as sources of stress. Persons with Panic Disorder often have a parent who has had similar symptoms. Some people with Panic Disorder have symptoms brought out by underlying medical problems, such as heart or thyroid conditions, for which they should see their doctor. An individual who develops Social Phobia, which is apparently much more common than had been realized, may have a childhood history of social constraint and shyness. People who have Panic Disorder or Social Phobia often have other anxiety and depressive disorders. For instance, more than half of people with Panic Disorder have also had Major Depressive Disorder.

Onset and Course

Panic Disorder and Agoraphobia most often begin between the late teens and mid-thirties. Social Phobia usually begins in the mid-teens, whereas many Specific Phobias begin in childhood.

Once Panic Disorder occurs, Agoraphobia can then occur at any point, although most often appearing in the first year if there are repeated panic attacks. Specific Phobias developing in childhood often clear up by themselves. However, Panic and Phobic Disorders in adult life tend not to resolve themselves. The longer the symptoms exist, the more effect they will have on a person's life and the harder it will be to effect change. Social Phobia may appear to go away, but the problem is often still there. For instance, the person who fears dating may be fine after marriage, only to have the problem recur after the death or divorce of the spouse. In all anxiety disorders, there is a risk of substance abuse as a way of self-treating symptoms.

Treatment

Self-Help. People with panic and phobic symptoms are often very private and are ashamed about their symptoms, so they endure them in painful silence. They can be helped a good deal by the many books about these syndromes that reveal that they are far from alone in having such symptoms and can also inform them about seeking help. One such book is *Triumph over Fear* by Jerilyn Ross and Rosalynn Carter. There is also a video produced by the American Psychiatric Association titled *Anxiety Disorders: New Diagnostic Issues*. Often persons with Panic Disorder and Agoraphobia are helped a great deal by joining self-help groups of others with the same types of symptoms who carry out feared activities together. Persons with Social Phobia are sometimes helped by support groups such as Dale Carnegie and Toastmasters. The Anxiety Disorders Association of America is a major advocacy organization.

Professional Help. People with Anxiety Disorders require treatment from experts to help them grasp the nature of their symptoms, the personal causes for them, how to recover and how to prevent symptoms from coming back in the future. When panic symptoms are acute and impair normal activities, prescribed drugs may be necessary.

Section 2: Obsessive-Compulsive Disorder

Doctor: What is it she does now? Look how she rubs her hands.

Gentlewoman: It is an accustomed action with her, to seem thus washing her
hands. I have known her to continue in this a quarter of an hour.

Lady Macbeth: Yet here's a spot . . . Out, damned spot! out I say! . . . What! will
these hands ne'er be clean?

William Shakespeare, Macbeth, 1606

What Is the Definition?

The word *obsess* comes from the Latin *obsidere*, "to beset" and *compulsion* comes from
the Latin *compulsus*, "to compel." A person with Obsessive-Compulsive Disorder
(OCD) is beset by unwanted thoughts or impulses and feels compelled to engage in
repetitive actions that have no practical purpose. Many people dwell at times on
upsetting thoughts and can have minor compulsive behaviors, but a diagnosis of
OCD is not made unless obsessions and compulsions cause marked distress, take up
a lot of time (more than one hour a day), or block daily routines such as school, work,
or friendships.

What Are the Symptoms?

Common types of obsessions are intrusive worries about being touched by
someone such as in shaking hands, possibly having hit someone while driving, or
having left home without locking up. A person can have fearful impulses that are
most often resisted, such as urges to curse loudly in front of others. There can be
great concern that everything in the home must be in its own very special location.
Compulsions involve repeated acts that cannot be resisted, such as hand washing,
checking if doors are locked, and repeating prayers over and over for hours, acts that
are carried on in order to reduce the extreme tension that builds up while trying to
resist the urges. Children may not know when their worries don't make sense,
whereas adults do know and yet feel compelled to have the thoughts and acts
anyway. People with OCD also frequently have other anxiety and depressive
disorders.

Who Is Affected?

A nationwide survey found that 2 percent of the population had OCD at some
point in 1990. OCD may occur more often in identical twins than in fraternal twins,
and it occurs equally in males and females, except in childhood where boys show
symptoms more often than girls. As for other Anxiety Disorders, there are complex
causes for OCD involving temperament and life events.

Onset and Course

OCD can begin in childhood but usually starts in the teen or early adult years. Its onset is most often gradual.

Most people with OCD develop a chronic illness that tends to cycle from periods when they have many symptoms to times with only a few; the symptoms are usually brought on by stress. Without expert help and after long-term failure to resist the thoughts and urges, the person may give in to them, no longer struggling, ending in a lifestyle that makes him or her a lasting prisoner of the obsessions and compulsions. This can result in isolation from others and chronic job failure.

Treatment

Self-Help. In most cases, self-help is not very useful for people with OCD, although reading about the disorder and researching what is said about it on the Internet can help a person feel less alone and perhaps push him or her to seek expert help. A major advocacy organization is the Obsessive Compulsive Foundation. A video about the disorder, *Children with OCD*, can be obtained from the American Psychiatric Association.

Professional Help. People with OCD require psychotherapy and often drugs from experts skilled in treating the disorder. As in all the Anxiety Disorders, it can be very helpful to work with an expert to learn about the nature of the condition, the events in one's life that led to problems in self-esteem and in relationships with others, and the kinds of steps required to decrease the symptoms. With regard to drug treatment, certain antidepressants and related drugs have been found to be helpful for many people with this disorder.

Section 3: Posttraumatic Stress Disorder

Extreme fear can neither fight nor fly.
William Shakespeare, *The Rape of Lucrece*, 1593–94

What Is the Definition?

The word *stress* comes from the Latin *stringere*, which means "to draw tight." The word *trauma* is Greek, meaning "hurt or wound." A person with Posttraumatic Stress Disorder (PTSD) has been "drawn tight" by severe stress symptoms as a result of being threatened with death or severe injury, or having witnessed another person being killed or threatened with death. To be given this diagnosis, the person must have major symptoms based on a trauma that caused extreme feelings of mortal fear or helplessness, with resulting problems in social, work, or other aspects of daily life.

What Are the Symptoms?

A person with PTSD has three types of symptoms. First, the trauma continues to recur in painful memories and dreams, with intense distress when exposed to something that reminds the individual of the event. Second, the person tries to avoid any thoughts, feelings, actions, places, or people that elicit such memories and may not even be able to recall key aspects of the trauma. There may be an associated loss of interests and a sensation of numbness about daily activities and events, along with a feeling of distance from other people, even to the extent of not being able to have feelings of affection for anyone. There may also be a sense of impending doom and an expectation of early death. Third, there are very troubling symptoms that can include poor sleep and concentration, feelings of crankiness and anger, and hypervigilance along with being easily startled. Children may become confused and agitated and may repeat the trauma in play, such as crashing toy cars when they have been in or seen a car crash.

Who Is Affected?

About one person in a hundred has this condition at some point during their lifetimes, and it occurs twice as often in females as in males. Some people can live through extreme traumas without developing PTSD, while others are very susceptible. It can occur in up to 30 percent of disaster victims. People who respond immediately to traumas by becoming numb or having strong avoidance symptoms are at higher risk for PTSD. It has been found that early life experiences can set the stage. Adult children of Holocaust survivors are more likely to develop PTSD after traumas, and one-third of persons with Borderline Personality Disorder also have PTSD (see chapter 15).

Onset and Course

PTSD can occur at any age. For children, sexual, physical, and emotional abuse can trigger PTSD, with or without clear threat of death or severe injury. Traumas that can be followed by PTSD include combat, rape, assault, domestic violence, kidnapping, torture, internment in a concentration camp, natural disasters, and life-threatening illness.

About half of those with PTSD recover within three months. Many others have symptoms that become chronic, sometimes resulting in joblessness or causing them to live almost as a hermit.

Treatment

Self-Help. A person who knows that he or she has PTSD can benefit from reading about the causes, symptoms, and paths to healing. It has been found that after a plane crash or other group disaster, survivors and involved parties can be helped by coming together and bonding. Bonding in supportive groups has also helped Vietnam and Gulf War veterans with PTSD. Powerful accounts of PTSD are found in Primo Levi's *Survival in Auschwitz: The Nazi Assault on Humanity* and William Styron's *Sophie's Choice*. The American Psychiatric Association has produced a video titled *Posttraumatic Stress Disorder*.

Professional Help. The sooner a person with PTSD symptoms seeks help from an expert, the more likely it is that the symptoms will last only a brief time. Psycho-therapy is almost always necessary, beginning with crisis intervention immediately after traumas, along with group support. Many people experience great guilt about the deaths of others and must be given guidance right away. Vulnerable people with childhood histories of trauma and loss may require longer-term intensive psycho-therapy. Acute symptoms may respond to drugs, chiefly antidepressants. Chronic PTSD that has lasted for many years is very hard to treat.

Section 4: Generalized Anxiety Disorder

For as children tremble and fear everything in the blind darkness, so we in the light sometimes fear what is no more to be feared than the things children in the dark hold in terror and imagine will come true.
Lucretius [Titus Lucretius Carus], *De Rerum Natura*, 99–55 B.C.

What Is the Definition?

The word *anxious* comes from the Latin *angere*, which means "to torment." In Generalized Anxiety Disorder (GAD), the person is tormented by undue anxiety, worry, and foreboding that has been going on for at least six months and that he or she cannot control. Everyone at times feels anxiety, but the diagnosis of GAD is made only when symptoms cause considerable distress or seriously hinder work, social, or other key aspects of daily living.

What Are the Symptoms?

A person with GAD feels restless or very uneasy, tires easily, has trouble concen-trating, and may lose track of his or her thoughts at times. There may be a feeling of crankiness as well. In addition, there are physical symptoms, such as tense, aching muscles and troubled sleep. This diagnosis is not made if the symptoms are part of some other disorder, such as panic states, phobias, or OCD.

Who Is Affected?

About 60 percent of people with this disorder are women, and there is a trend for family members to experience anxiety more often than in other families. About five of every one hundred people have had an episode of significant GAD in their lifetimes.

Onset and Course

Many people with GAD say that they have felt anxious and have been worriers all of their lives. In fact, about half of those with the disorder began to have definite symptoms in childhood or their teens. Children with GAD tend to be conforming, to have a need to be perfect, to be unsure of themselves, and to require extra approval and reassurance. GAD tends to become chronic if the person does not receive expert help.

A person who seems to have GAD must be asked about medical illness or drug abuse and may need a physical examination and laboratory testing, because illness as well as drugs may cause symptoms such as those of GAD.

Treatment

Self-Help. Persons with milder forms of GAD can often be helped by confiding in friends, getting comfort from them as well as good practical advice about their excessive worries. Reading about anxiety, and learning from books that they are far from alone in having such symptoms, can be quite reassuring. The character of Blanche DuBois in Tennessee Williams's *A Streetcar Named Desire* and the lead characters in Woody Allen's *Annie Hall* illustrate chronic anxiety and its effects.

Professional Help. Very often stress, abuse, and loss in childhood and the teen years, as well as other prior painful life events, are the background for a present-day vulnerability to stress; in such cases, people require professional help from experts. Since a person may be confused about the meaning of the prior life experiences, and may have even learned to blame himself or herself wrongly, it is necessary for the expert to have had thorough training and experience in detecting key aspects of a person's unique history and in helping the patient to understand them. With reassurance and self-knowledge, people can improve greatly and learn to deal successfully with stress in the future. In the case of severe symptoms, there are many antianxiety drugs that can be used temporarily, and because depression often occurs along with GAD, some patients may require both antianxiety and antidepressant drugs.

L. Park

Chapter 7
Somatoform Disorders

Soma is the Greek word for "body," and *somatoform* describes a mental illness that presents itself in the form of an illness of the body. It can take a number of patterns, but a diagnosis of this kind should be made only after a physical illness has been ruled out by a thorough medical workup.

Section 1: Somatization Disorder

What is good we remember. What is bad we feel.

Jewish Folk Saying

What Is the Definition?

The person's mental distress is felt as physical and believed to be physical, though its cause is not physical.

What Are the Symptoms?

Often Somatization has many different symptoms. The symptoms do not fit any known disease or syndrome or are far in excess of what would be expected based on a physical exam or lab tests. There also tend to be symptoms at many different sites. The complaints may be of pain or other trouble, for instance, nausea, bloating, vomiting, diarrhea, or irregular menstrual periods. With this disorder, the symptoms are not feigned or produced intentionally. Persons with Anxiety, Panic, and Mood Disorders may have somatic symptoms, but the somatic symptoms begin after the onset of the mental states and the focus is not mainly on the body symptoms.

Who Is Affected?

Women are affected with Somatization Disorder more often than men. It begins before age thirty and often appears first in adolescence. Menstrual problems may be one of the first symptoms. There may be a family history of Somatization Disorder on the female side and of Antisocial Personality Disorder and substance abuse on the male side.

Onset and Course

Although stress starts the cascade of somatic symptoms, cultural factors appear to play a part in this unique response and shape its features. The most serious risk is that a grave medical illness will be missed because it was decided (without a thorough medical workup) that the symptoms do not have a physical cause; it should not be assumed that all new symptoms are explained by this diagnosis and therefore do not require further study. But not making the diagnosis in a timely way carries the danger that a person with this disorder will be treated with sundry drugs for an "organic" illness that does not exist, thus exposing an individual to the hazards of taking drugs they do not need and should not be taking (e.g., adverse side effects, substance abuse). A further risk is that the family will spend much money on a fruitless search for a cause that cannot be found outside the mind.

Treatment

Self-Help. A person should have respect for the fact that mental states can affect the body and even cause symptoms in diverse organ systems.

Professional Help. A thorough medical workup is a must, because without one, true physical illness cannot be ruled out. Somatization Disorder is a diagnosis of *exclusion*. Once made, though, a psychiatric specialist should assess the personal, social, school, or work factors in the patient's life and suggest a treatment approach. Treatment may include one or more of these elements: psychotherapy, medication, physical therapy, and changing the environment.

Section 2: Conversion Disorder

Between the idea
And the reality
Between the motion
And the act
Falls the shadow.

T. S. Eliot, *The Hollow Men*, 1925

What Is the Definition?

To *convert* means "to turn into" and *conversion* means "turning from one state into another," for instance, water turning from liquid into ice. It is in this sense that the word is used in this disorder—that is, specific ideas (not just "distress") are turned from a mental domain into a physical symptom. Some of Freud's first cases were of this nature.

What Are the Symptoms?

The symptoms of Conversion Disorder are more limited in type than those for Somatization Disorder and only involve systems of the body that are normally thought to be under conscious control or awareness. That would, for example, include paralysis of an arm or leg, sudden blindness, deafness, numbness, loss of balance, or a lump in the throat, but *not* stomach pain, intestinal cramps, bladder urgency, menstrual pain, or the like.

These symptoms would be very grave if they were early signs of real organic disease, but if nothing is confirmed, they point to profound psychic problems. Though the diagnosis is made by ruling out true somatic disease, doctors often find clues to this diagnosis by the fact that the symptoms do not follow known nerve pathways or a known disease process. The patient may show *la belle indifférence*, French for a "beautiful lack of concern," perhaps aware (though not consciously) that there is no danger from the presumed dreadful symptoms.

Who Is Affected?

Conversion Disorder may run in families and is more common among women than men. The illness is more likely to occur in places or among people who have less knowledge about health and disease processes; it is more common in rural locales and among the poor. In earlier times, organic causes were found in 25 to 50 percent of patients who were given the diagnosis in error. In more recent studies, the incidence is much lower, perhaps because doctors and patients are more aware of the disorder and techniques for probing the body have improved.

Onset and Course

The most frequent age of onset is between ten and thirty-five years, but it can occur at any age. Freud's case of Fraulein Elisabeth von R in the *Standard Edition* is one of the best examples of such a case (see appendix B). In children under ten, gait problems and "seizures" tend to predominate. The disorder is often found under states of extreme stress, for instance, war or the death of a person significant to the patient.

The risk here is that a thorough workup may not be performed and a real physical illness missed. The disorder will recur in 20 to 25 percent of patients within one year. Some patients later will show the full range of symptoms of Somatization Disorder described above.

Treatment

Self-Help. The person should be aware that mental conditions can cause somatic symptoms. Having a trusted physician who knows the family or patient is very helpful.

Professional Help. The course of illness is usually short and may improve quickly when no fatal disease is found. If treatment is needed, it would involve the same techniques outlined under Somatization Disorder.

Section 3: Pain Disorder

The two foes of human happiness are pain and boredom.
                    Arthur Schopenhauer, "Personality; or, What a Man Is," 1851

What Is the Definition?

Pain comes from the Latin word that means "punishment" or "torment." There is often a feeling of torment that surrounds and invests the sensation of "hurt" caused by harm to the body.

What Are the Symptoms?

There are two subtypes here: one where medical illness plays little or no part in the Pain Disorder and the other where it is a large partner. If mental factors play no role and the pain is related only to an organic disease, this diagnosis is not used. "Acute" is used for pain lasting less than six months and "chronic" for pain of six months or longer. This diagnosis is used if doctors judge that mental factors play a role in the onset, degree, or waxing and waning of pain. There must also be other symptoms, such as the pain becoming a major focus of the person's life; heavy use or abuse of medications; the pain triggering problems with spouse or children; the person not working or going to school because of the pain. *La belle indifference* is *never* present.

Who Is Affected?

This disorder may happen at any time, but it tends to be seen more commonly in the fourth and fifth decades of life. It occurs in both sexes but more often in women than men. Women particularly suffer more migraines and musculoskeletal symptoms. Pain Disorder is more frequent in people working in blue-collar-type jobs and often may be job-related. It is more common in families where others have this disorder; Depressive Disorders, Anxiety Disorders, and Substance Abuse Disorders are also more common in these families.

Onset and Course

Personal factors play a part in the development of Pain Disorder, but also in different ethnic groups pain may have different meanings. Loss of job and a decline in income, as well as family problems, often occur with this disorder. Doctors may prescribe opiates and benzodiazepines, which can result in dependence or abuse. Where pain is tied to a fatal illness, there is a higher risk of suicide. Lack of motion due to the pain may lead to increased depression and increased fatigue levels. Acute pain is more often linked to anxiety disorders and chronic pain to depressive disorders.

Treatment

Self-Help. Resistance to letting the pain become *the* factor that dictates how a person lives his or her life (not turning "hurt" into "torment") is crucial to getting back one's mental health. Regular activities and schedules are essential. Literary sources that deal with the theme of pain include Aeschylus's *Prometheus Bound* and Percy Bysshe Shelley's *Prometheus Unbound*.

Professional. Having a trusted doctor with whom one can discuss options that one might pursue is very important. It is common for acute pain to resolve quickly. Searching for the "cure" for chronic pain, though, is often pursuing a phantom. "Pain management" thus becomes the goal. A specialist can assess the factors in the patient's life and suggest a useful approach. It may include psychotherapy, medication, or a special program that involves physical therapy and group methods, or some blend of these. Improvement of function and quality of life, rather than full pain relief, must be the goal.

Section 4: Hypochondriasis

How sickness enlarges the dimensions of a man's self to himself.
Charles Lamb, "The Convalescent," 1833

What Is the Definition?

Here, the root word is not helpful and merely refers to the body site thought by the Greeks to cause this syndrome (i.e., below the rib cage and above the belly button). Hypochondriasis is the anguish about a grave physical illness where there is no basis in fact for thinking one has it.

What Are the Symptoms?

Although most people might become upset over minor changes in body sensations, if those changes do not progress, or if medical help is sought and results do not reveal disease, the normal person is relieved. But in persons with Hypochondriasis, the concern about health persists in excess for at least six months even with proof to the contrary. Indeed, this is a group of patients who may "doctor shop," hoping to find someone who will confirm their belief. They strongly oppose offers of mental health treatment. Social ties can become strained, they may miss time at work, and they can end up invalids. Woody Allen has often played such a person in films.

Who Is Affected?

Males and females are affected equally often. The disorder usually begins in early adulthood, and the course is chronic with periods of being better and worse. In a large, general medical practice, estimates can be as high as almost 10 percent of patients seen.

Onset and Course

Some things that have been thought to be linked to the onset of Hypochondriasis are a major illness in childhood or a serious, perhaps fatal, illness in a family member. Reading or hearing about a disease has also been known to suggest it in some people (e.g., medical students).

The risks here are that doctors may not treat symptoms with sufficient concern when there *is* an organic disease. Indeed, after frequent visits with similar complaints, an illness may be missed because it was not pursued (the "crying wolf" case). These people may become shunned both at home and at work, as they weary others with their constant complaints. They miss time at work, which may lead to losing a job.

Treatment

Self-Help. Keeping an open mind about the effect of mental states on physical ones is helpful, because it is known that the psyche can have profound effects on the body.

Professional Help. Having a general medical physician whom the patient trusts enough to consult and who knows the patient is vital. The focus of mental health care is not cure of a somatic disease but trying to maintain function, as with Pain Disorder, discussed above.

Section 5: Body Dysmorphic Disorder

For of the soul the body form doth take:
For soul is form, and doth the body make.

Edmund Spenser, *Hymn in Honor of Beauty*, 1596

What Is the Definition?

Morphe means "form" and *dys* means "bad," so this is a mental disorder where a person tends to focus on a defect in the form of the body. It was also known in the past as "dysmorphophobia."

What Are the Symptoms?

Complaints by persons with Body Dysmorphic Disorder often involve slight flaws, of face or figure well within the normal spectrum, that are blown up and focused on and cause the sufferer great anguish. Affected people may spend hours daily thinking about the "defect" to the point that it controls their lives. There may be frequent mirror checking or use of magnifying glasses, and they may even install special lights. The person may think that others are talking about or mocking them because of it. They may even avoid school, dating, or job interviews because of it. If the belief is bizarre and held with intense conviction, it may be called "Delusional Disorder, Somatic Type."

Who Is Affected?

Body Dysmorphic Disorder often begins in the teenage years and appears equally often among men and women. Those affected are likely to be unmarried. A survey of college students indicated that more than half were preoccupied with some aspect of their appearance. The estimate of the prevalence of this disorder in plastic surgery and dermatology practices is on the order of 6 to 15 percent of patients. Cultural factors may play a part.

Onset and Course

This illness may range in degree from mild to severe. In the latter group, persons may be housebound because of it or even make a suicide attempt. Some people have repeated plastic surgery on the same sites without ever being satisfied and can spend a great deal of money doing so. They may avoid school, dating, job interviews, and contact with other people due to their distress. No reassurance seems to help.

Treatment

Self-Help. It is vital not to give in to the desire to avoid others until one is "perfect." One must also form a grace for living with one's own and others' shortcomings. There are a number of literary works that deal with this subject, including Edmund Rostand's *Cyrano de Bergerac* and Hans Christian Andersen's *The Ugly Duckling.*

Professional Help. There is a French saying, "*Chacun a son gout,*" which means "Each to his own taste." Cosmetic surgery exists so that patients can achieve their idea of beauty even though they were not born with it. But this shades off into a mental disorder when enough repair of an imperfection can never be achieved or when the distress at the flaw is too great and causes the person to be unable to function in society. Then expert psychiatric help should be sought.

T. Allen

Chapter 8
Factitious Disorders

Oh, what a tangled web we weave,
When first we practice to deceive!

Sir Walter Scott, *Lochinvar*, 1808

What Is the Definition?

Factitious comes from the Latin word *facere*, meaning to "make" (as in manufacture) something, in this case an illness that is *not* produced by nature that permits the person to assume a sick role.

What Are the Symptoms?

A person with a factitious disorder causes an illness in himself or herself, for instance, by taking anticoagulants so blood will be found in the urine. The person may feign symptoms of an illness, such as a grand mal seizure. It is not "malingering," because it is not being used as a means to an end (e.g., to avoid a trial). The goal is simply to appear sick and thus receive care, sympathy and concern.

There are three subtypes of patients: those with mostly physical signs and symptoms; those with mostly mental signs and symptoms; and those with a combination. There is a related syndrome in which an illness is induced in someone else, usually a child, and the parent or caretaker presents the child to a doctor with the "illness." In this case, the parent causes the illness by giving the child a drug or perhaps puts blood in the urine, and the parent-child bond prevents the child from telling.

Who Is Affected?

Factitious disorders are most often first seen in young adults. They are more common in males than females, but it remains a rare disorder. Factors that may play a part are a history of a major illness in childhood in the patient or in a family member, presence of other physical or mental ailments, or a job in the medical or hospital field.

Onset and Course

There may be only one or two discrete events, but more commonly this disorder tends to become a chronic pattern. Patients often flee the doctor or hospital when their "illness" is correctly diagnosed, leaving Against Medical Advice. As a result, they do not get any real insight into why they engage in this behavior. Many are "loners" and tend to simply repeat the pattern with a new doctor or hospital. They do often succeed in getting doctors to operate on them or to give them drugs, and they may suffer from needless adverse outcomes as a result. These patients can provoke a very profound medical illness by taking a risky drug to induce a factitious illness. Some get hooked on drugs to relieve pain complaints that are feigned. They are rarely able to enjoy a stable work or family life, because anyone who cares for the patient is destined to feel exploited. There is a subgroup diagnosed as "Munchausen Syndrome" patients (after the famous Baron Munchausen); their entire lives revolve around trying to get admitted to hospitals. "Munchausen by Proxy" refers to those parents who induce the "illness" in the child as described above.

Treatment

Self-Help. Having a trusted doctor in whom one can confide may avert the need to seek support for an illness that is feigned. Also, having a wide social circle makes it likely that one will have some person with whom one can share things.

Professional Help. Unfortunately not much is known about these patients, because they tend to run away once the diagnosis is made. Yet if they could engage with a mental health specialist, they would have the chance to learn why they follow this pattern and could, perhaps, change it.

T. Allen

Chapter 9
Dissociative Disorders

The word *dissociation* comes from the Latin prefix *dis-*, which means "to be apart from," and from the Latin word *sociare*, which means "to join." One who dissociates is distant from or apart from the self or from one's sense of self. Thus, people in a dissociative state may not recall certain facts or remember certain past events, or they may not know where they are at a certain time, or how they got there, or who they are as a person. Dissociative disorders are divided into four major groups: Dissociative Amnesia, Dissociative Fugue, Dissociative Identity Disorder (DID), and Depersonalization Disorder.

Section 1: Dissociative Amnesia

It is the distance of not listening, the malady of not marking that I am troubled withal.

William Shakespeare, *King Henry IV*, 1598

What Is the Definition?

The word *amnesia* comes from the Greek word *amnesia*, which means "forgetfulness." People with Dissociative Amnesia cannot recall certain facts. Dissociative Amnesia differs from Amnestic Disorder (see chapter 2), as the former is brought on by events evoking threatening or painful memories in contrast to the latter, which is brought on by acute or chronic medical disorders.

What Are the Symptoms?

Persons with Dissociative Amnesia may forget who they are, who another person is, events that occurred in the past, or previously known facts. The events not recalled are often of a painful and stressful nature, such as in wartime or with a car crash. This illness may also occur when one has hurt oneself, has been hurt by someone else, has hurt another person, or has seen a death occur. These stressful events, which one "forgets," may pertain to a certain past time and place. The event may not be recalled at all or may be recalled only in part. A person with amnesia may also be depressed, appear to be in a trance, regress back in time to early childhood behavior, or perhaps have a certain kind of memory loss, such as forgetting how to do simple math problems. These patients are often highly hypnotizable.

Who Is Affected?

Dissociative Amnesia may occur at any age. Very little is known about how often and in which groups of people it occurs.

Onset and Course

Amnesias may be hard to assess in children. They appear mostly in the teen or adult years and seem to be caused by stressful events at any time from childhood onward. Amnesia may appear all of a sudden in a stressful situation and then vanish just as quickly when the person leaves the situation. In chronic cases, the recall of past painful events sometimes occurs on its own.

The person may forget a span of time from a few months to a few years. While only a single amnestic event may be spoken about, most patients "forget" two or more such past events. If amnesia is caused by a single trauma, it is easier for the patient eventually to recall the event and put it behind them. If these traumas have occurred more often, as with abuse in children, a more chronic amnesia usually remains and can have a severe effect on their personal, social, school, and work life.

Treatment

Self-Help. Reading books or pamphlets on this topic may help to learn more about how best to avoid stressful events that may set off the symptoms of Dissociative Amnesia.

Professional Help. Through psychotherapy, the patient can be helped to recall past events that have been forgotten. Hypnosis and medication can also be used to help the patient recall forgotten past events. Sometimes inpatient or day care treatment is needed.

Section 2: Dissociative Fugue

What way shall I fly? Infinite wrath and infinite despair?
. . . and in the lowest deep, a lower deep . . .
to which the hell I suffer seems a heaven.

John Milton, *Paradise Lost*, 1667

What Is the Definition?

The word *fugue* is French and comes from the Latin *fugere*, which means "to flee." The person in a fugue state flees from one place, such as home or work, and is found later in a distant place, not knowing how or why he or she got there.

What Are the Symptoms?

The individual travels to a distant, strange place with no clear reason for doing so, and often without being able to recall even going there. At the new place, his or her actions often do not seem to draw notice from others at first. However, the fugue victim may finally become aware of what has happened and call family or friends for help in getting back home, or may be picked up by the police because of confusion or amnesia and taken to a hospital emergency room for care. A fugue state normally lasts only a short time, but it may also go on for many weeks or months, during which time the person is out of touch with home and family. Sometimes, he or she may even take on a new name.

Who Is Affected?

In some cultures, "running" or "fleeing" in an altered state is more common. The Mesketo people of Honduras and Nicaragua call it "trisi siknis," and the Western Pacific peoples call it "amok," both of which may fit the diagnosis for Dissociative Fugue. It has been reported that about 0.2 percent of the general population has had at least one fugue state, and this number may increase in times of war or natural disaster.

Onset and Course

Fugue states appear suddenly and are brought on mostly in the adult years by severe life stresses, such as losing a loved one or viewing a fearful or painful event. Most people recover quickly from these fugue events, but some cases linger much longer, requiring more active treatment for many months.

Treatment

Self-Help. A person prone to fugue states may learn about this illness and the stressful events that may set off a tendency to flee. The individual may then learn to avoid such events.

Professional Help. Psychotherapy may help the patient recall the past events that brought on the fugue state. Hypnosis and medication are also helpful in this effort. Psychotherapy may include both one-to-one and group therapy.

Section 3: Dissociative Identity Disorder (Formerly Multiple Personality Disorder)

And long we try in vain to speak and act our hidden self
And what we do and say is eloquent as well
But tis not true.

                    Matthew Arnold, *The Buried Life*, 1862

What Is the Definition?

The word *identity* comes from the Latin word *indentitas*, which means "the same." In this illness, a person's sense of sameness or oneness, or sense of self, is broken into two or more distinct identities or altered personality states.

What Are the Symptoms?

The major feature of Dissociative Identity Disorder (DID) is that the person has two or more distinct states of self that may alter the person's actions, feelings, or speech during a certain period of time. One's personality or "altered state of mind" may not recognize past events that another personality or altered state does recall. These personalities may have distinct names, actions, and memories of past events, which sometimes may suggest how they came into being. These altered states may be frightened, angry, depressed, or violent or self-hurting in their actions. They may be any age and either gender. For example, a grown woman may all of a sudden display the actions, speech, and sense of self of a little boy. This "little boy" may continue to be present for several minutes or several hours and may perhaps talk about being hurt by "Daddy" when "he" was three years old. These altered states appear mostly when a person feels threatened by certain life events.

Who Is Affected?

Over the last few years, DID has been diagnosed much more often than in the past. Some experts think the increase in diagnosis is due to a greater awareness of its symptoms and its causes which include abuse in childhood; others think that the increase is really due to patients being encouraged "to recall past childhood abuses" and being given suggestions of symptoms of the illness they might have. The diagnosis is made three to four times more often in women than in men. It is more often seen in people who had a parent with the illness than in the public at large. The illness may be diagnosed at any age.

Onset and Course

People with DID often report a history of some physical, sexual, or verbal abuse as a child six years old or younger, usually lasting many months. The onset of altered states is sudden, generally caused by a stressful event that threatens the person. Sometimes, two or more altered states may blend to give an even more complex picture. The average number of altered states is seven to eight, but the mode is twelve.

Often, at least one personality is very angry and may turn that anger onto itself. Suicidal acts are common. Most patients have headaches and gastrointestinal problems. The changes in behavior are viewed by others "as if you're another person," not realizing the truth of the matter. People with DID often suffer from other mental illnesses, such as Bipolar II Disorder, Posttraumatic Stress Disorder, Borderline Personality Disorder, and substance abuse. Likewise, they often suffer from many physical illnesses.

Treatment

Self-Help. Both reading books about this illness and being in DID self-help groups can help the patient and family better understand the complex nature of this disorder and cope with its symptoms. The Sidran Foundation offers training, brochures, and books about trauma and dissociation and refers patients to local self-help groups and clinicians. *Multiple Personality Disorder from the Inside Out,* edited by Barry Cohen, Esther Giller, and Lynn W. (a patient), includes vignettes from 146 adults diagnosed with DID. *My Mom Is Different* by Debora Sessions is a picture book for children with a parent who has a dissociative disorder.

Professional Help. A proper diagnosis is often very hard to make, because the patient may be unaware of the illness as such, may purposely hide the symptoms, or may have other physical and mental illnesses that can distract a doctor from the DID. Psychotherapy, both in groups and on a one-to-one basis, is the treatment of choice. Sometimes hypnosis and medications are helpful in reducing some of the symptoms or some of the other illnesses. Sometimes inpatient and day care treatment may be needed.

Section 4: Depersonalization Disorder

Where are we? And why are we? Of what scene; the actors or spectators?
                              Percy Bysshe Shelley, *Adonais*, 1821

What Is the Definition?

The word *depersonalization* comes from the Latin prefix *de-*, which means "away from," and the Latin word *persona*, which means "person" or "self." Thus, depersonalization refers to people moving away from themselves and losing touch with their feelings as if they were robots or characters in a play.

What Are the Symptoms?

A person with Depersonalization Disorder feels detached from him- or herself and feels "unreal," as if acting in or watching a play. A change in body feeling, such as numbness, may be present. For example, a patient may feel estranged, "out of touch," as if from another place, even another planet. "I feel like I'm a Martian," said one patient to his doctor, even though he knew that these strange feelings were unreal.

Who Is Affected?

Certain cultures and religions voluntarily utilize trance and meditation states, but this is quite different from the acute onset of trance states that occur under stress. Women are said to have Depersonalization Disorder twice as often as males. However, up to 50 percent of healthy people have had one or two short depersonalization episodes while under acute stress. In life-threatening danger, one-third of the people involved depersonalize. Nearly 40 percent of patients treated in mental hospitals or on psychiatric units depersonalize.

Onset and Course

The symptoms of Depersonalization Disorder appear when a person feels threatened and may last for only a few moments, or up to several years. They may also occur and recur over time. However, people generally do not complain about this illness. Rather, a person more often comes to treatment because he or she feels depressed or anxious. The onset of the depersonalization illness is sudden, touched off by some remark or event that threatens the person. The symptoms often accompany other mental illnesses, such as depression, anxiety, panic attacks, as well as certain physical illnesses.

Over time, the person comes to learn that these sensations, the sense of numbness and distance from oneself, are a serious problem. A person's social life or achievements at work or in school can be markedly lessened by these depersonalized states of mind.

Treatment

Self-Help. People can read pamphlets or books which help explain Depersonalization Disorder. See the national referral sources and books mentioned in the previous section, "Dissociative Identity Disorder."

Professional Help. Psychotherapy is the primary treatment to help the patient understand what was so fearful as to cause depersonalization and how best to work through the feelings and other symptoms of this disorder. Hypnosis and medication are also helpful in getting the patient to feel less frightened and more at peace.

M. Liebman

Chapter 10
Sexual and Gender Identity Disorders

There are three major groups of sexual and gender identity disorders: Sexual Dysfunction, Paraphilia, and Gender Identity Disorder.

Section 1: Sexual Dysfunction

When we will, they won't;
When we don't want to, they [women]
Want to exceedingly.

Terence, Eunuchus, ca. 190–159 B.C.

What Is the Definition?

The word *sex* is derived from the Latin word *sexus*, which means "separate," and refers to a state of being "separate" as either a male or a female. Sex can also refer to an action, such as "having sex." People with sexual dysfunctions have problems in the response cycle of the sexual act itself.

What Are the Symptoms?

The response cycle in sex can be broken down into four distinct phases: (1) the desire for sex; (2) a sense of excitement, pleasure, and certain bodily changes during the sex act; (3) a peaking of pleasure, release of tension, and rhythmic muscle movement, that is, orgasm; and (4) the release and sense of well-being following sex. Each phase has its own distinct mental disorders:

Phase 1: A decrease in daydreams and desire for sex.
Phase 2: A female not being able to attain and maintain excitement so as to reach orgasm, or a male not being able to attain and maintain an erect penis so as to have an orgasm or please the female partner.
Phase 3: A female not being able to achieve orgasm in a suitable length of time or not having an orgasm at all despite a normal excitement phase, or a male not being able to have an orgasm at all or within a suitable time despite contact between the male and female sex organs, or a rapid onset of penile discharge and orgasm shortly after sex begins, which

lessens the woman's pleasure.

Phase 4: Pain during or after sex in either a male or female, not due to a medical condition, or a spasm of the muscles that surround the outer third of the vagina when the sex act begins, not due to a general medical condition.

Sexual dysfunction may also be caused by a general medical condition, such as diabetes, spinal cord injury; or by substance use that can cause any of the above symptoms.

Who Is Affected?

Sexual functioning is very sensitive to religious teachings, ethnic and cultural mores, and social background. Each of these affects one's expectations from sex and how one behaves toward the other person, as well as how one feels after the sex act. Another factor is gender; in many cultures, men are supposed to be "macho" and women more hesitant and demure. Finally, aging may be a factor that diminishes desire and performance, especially in men.

Although this subject has been widely researched, sexual dysfunction studies vary greatly. One comprehensive study for adults aged eighteen to fifty-nine produced the following data about dysfunction:

	% of men	% of women
pain during intercourse	3	15
orgasm problem	10	25
hypoactive desire	—	33
arousal problem	—	20
premature ejaculation	27	—
erection problems	10	—

Onset and Course

Symptoms of sexual dysfunction may come on quickly or slowly. Mental factors may be the cause of the problem, or a general medical condition or drug problem may combine with the mental problem. A general medical or substance or drug problem alone might account for most of these symptoms.

These symptoms may persist or recur. They may be lifelong or acquired after a phase of normal function. They may occur consistently, or they may occur in a limited context of a certain place, a partner, or arousal foreplay. One or more of these symptoms may occur at some time in almost everyone's life for a short period of time. Older people often show less interest in sex, men more so than women, but this decline with age varies greatly. Problems with sexual function may also be seen in other mental illnesses, including depression, anxiety, or psychosis.

Treatment

Self-Help. If sexual dysfunction symptoms appear rather quickly, a person might think about any mental changes toward his or her work, sex partner, or other issues in life that may have brought on the changes in sexual functioning. These problems may have an effect on the sexual act. The Impotence Information Center offers help in terms of information about sexual dysfunction. The book *Becoming Orgasmic* by Julia Heiman and Joseph Lopiccolo may also be helpful.

Professional Help. Treatment for any physical causes of dysfunction should be carried out as needed. Medications can lessen the symptoms of anxiety or may improve male potency. Psychotherapy on a one-to-one basis or couples therapy may lessen the symptoms. Sex education, such as learning new ways to be physically involved with one's sex partner, may also be helpful.

Section 2: Paraphilia

Breathes there a man with hide so tough
Who says two sexes aren't enough.

Samuel Hoffenstein, *Love Songs #3*, 1928

What Is the Definition?

The word *paraphilia* comes from the Latin prefix *para* which means "alongside of," and the Latin word *philia*, which means "love." People with this illness have interests in sex that parallel but are not the same as the normal love interests or actions.

What Are the Symptoms?

People with paraphilia have daydreams, urges, actions, or concerns about sex that involves objects that are not human, perverse pleasures, such as hurting or being hurt by one's sex partner, or having sex with children or unconsenting adults. Paraphilia would be diagnosed if these thoughts or actions continue for six months of more. There are at least eight diagnostic groupings within the paraphilias:

- Exhibitionism—Exposing one's sex organs to someone who does not expect it, sometimes in public.

- Fetishism—Needing nonhuman objects, such as stockings, brassieres, boots, or shoes, to be part of the sex act. This category does not include cross-dressing.
- Frotteurism—Touching or rubbing against someone who does not consent to it. This often occurs in a busy, crowded place, such as a bus.
- Pedophilia—Someone over sixteen years old being involved in a sexual act with someone thirteen years or younger.
- Sexual Masochism—Needing to be shamed, beaten, bound, or made to suffer in a real or pretend way, with or by a sex partner or by oneself alone as part of the sex act.
- Sexual Sadism—Needing daydreams, urges, or real acts of inflicting mental or physical pain on the sex partner, who may or may not consent to the beating or abuse.
- Transvestite Fetishism—Needing to wear clothes of the other gender. This behavior is described only in heterosexual males. Sexual masochism may be seen along with this illness.
- Voyeurism—Secretly watching a person, usually a stranger, disrobe, become naked, and perhaps become involved in the sex act. This secret "peeping" is part of the patient's need to become aroused and have an orgasm.

Who Is Affected?

Males comprise almost exclusively seven of the eight groups of paraphilias, and in the one group where women do appear, Sexual Masochism, they are outnumbered by men twenty to one. The mores and practices of one culture or religion may define certain sexual behavior as deviant, as another defines the behavior acceptable. Agreement on what is "deviant" is not always easy to achieve.

Onset and Course

Most adults with paraphilias have had these symptoms for many years, many having been involved with perverse sex play since childhood or their teen years and often having been seduced by older children or adults. They need these daydreams, fantasies, or objects to become aroused. Sometimes, these perverse acts occur only at certain times or in certain places, which may remind the person of past painful events. The person is otherwise able at other times or places to function in a normal fashion. Paraphilias are mostly against the law. People engaging in them can be arrested or lose their jobs or have their marriages break up.

Treatment

Self-Help. People with paraphilias are rarely moved to change or stop their actions on their own despite the awful legal risk they take. Most seek help because they are anxious or depressed or are forced to get treatment by the legal system. A national referral and educational group, which also collects nationwide data about paraphilias, is the Safer Society.

Professional Help. Clinics exist that focus on helping patients with paraphilias. These clinics are often part of a medical school or legal/court system. Group therapy that aids the patients to learn new ways of coping with these inner urges, daydreams, and actions can be helpful. Medications can help the patients both by decreasing their desires and excitement for perverse pleasures and by decreasing their symptoms, such as being anxious or depressed.

Section 3: Gender Identity Disorder

She is a gay man trapped in a woman's body.

Boy George and Spencer Bright,
Take It Like a Man: The Autobiography of Boy George, 1995

What Is the Definition?

The word *gender* comes from the Latin word *genus*, meaning "birth kind." People with Gender Identity Disorder wish to be members of the other "kind" and are constantly discomforted with their own gender, often feeling that the birth sex is not correct.

What Are the Symptoms?

Little boys who develop Gender Identity Disorder may prefer playing with little girls rather than with other boys, or may prefer girl's clothes to boy's clothes. They may draw pictures of pretty girls or play with female dolls, such as Barbie, and avoid rough-and-tumble games with boys. Some boys express their wish to be a girl and in rare cases state their disgust with their penis. Little girls with this syndrome may strongly resist female-type clothes or actions. Their heroes are strong males, such as Batman. They prefer boys as playmates and enjoy running and contact sports rather than playing with dolls. Adults with this illness try to live as the other gender. Many dress in clothes and act the social role of the other gender. Some males utilize makeup, hormones, and shaving to help pass themselves off to others as being females. Sometimes plastic surgery to change facial features or sexual organs is carried out. Teenagers with this syndrome may either act as children and prefer cross-sex roles in games, or act as adults and cross-dress. They are more guarded in their feelings about cross-dressing, and their families are typically quite upset at their actions or ideas.

Who Is Affected?

In some small European countries, the data indicate that one male per thirty thousand adult males and one female per one hundred thousand adult females pursue surgery for sex reassignment. In child clinics, boys are referred for evaluation of these symptoms five times more often than girls. In adult clinics, there are two to three times more males than females. This difference in gender numbers, however, may reflect that women who cross-identify are far more accepted by their peers and society at large than men who cross-identify. Likewise in children, a "tomboy" girl is far more accepted than a "sissy" boy.

Onset and Course

Gender Identity Disorder in children is usually diagnosed between ages two and four. By adult age, three-quarters of the children who were given this diagnosis no longer have it, but they are homosexual or bisexual. The other one-quarter of the children with the diagnosis grow up to have a normal gender identity. In adults, two forms of cross-dressing are seen: those who as children or teenagers began to cross-dress and simply do so as adults, and those who began to cross-dress in later life.

People with this syndrome mostly become "loners," either by their own choice or by being rejected by others. Males who act in a feminine manner or wear women's clothes often upset other males who reject, threaten, or even hurt them. Women with this syndrome have fewer problems with their friends.

Treatment

Self-Help. Most people with Gender Identity Disorder come for treatment because they are depressed, anxious, or very lonely. Reading books about this illness may help the patient to address it. Support groups can also be useful.

Professional Help. Psychotherapy and medicine may help relieve certain symptoms and reduce stress and harmful actions. Sometimes these patients seek surgery to change their sexual organs.

M. Liebman

Chapter 11
Eating Disorders

There are two main Eating Disorders: Anorexia Nervosa and Bulimia Nervosa. They refer to certain eating patterns that can produce grave illness and even death but where there are no physical causes for them.

Section 1: Anorexia Nervosa

O' that this too, too solid flesh would melt,
Thaw and resolve itself into a dew;
Or that the Everlasting had not fix'd
His canon 'gainst self-slaughter!

William Shakespeare, *Hamlet*, 1600

What Is the Definition?

Anorexia, from the Greek, means "lacking desire for food," and *nervosa* means "nerves"; hence, the syndrome refers to someone who lacks a desire for food because of "nerves." It is not really a loss of desire for food, but rather a situation in which the person perceives it to be in his or her interest to lose weight, even when it poses a profound threat to life.

What Are the Symptoms?

Symptoms of Anorexia include a refusal to stay above even the lowest recommended limits of body weight, fear of gaining weight even though it would merely be a return to normal weight, and a sense that the body is "fat" even when it is extremely thin. Females may stop having menses. The disorder involves not the loss of desire for food but a relentless rigid control of food intake so that the body remains in a depleted state. It can progress to purging and drastic exercise. Concern about being fat may be attached to the whole body or to parts of it—buttocks, stomach, thighs. Usually, family members bring the person in to the doctor, as the ill do not recognize the danger they have put themselves into. There are two subtypes of Anorexia: Restricting (diet) Type and the Binge Eating/Purging Type. The names are descriptive. There may be abnormal lab findings in many systems because of the lack of food, and there are many physical signs and symptoms.

Who Is Affected?

This syndrome rarely begins before puberty or after age forty, and 90 percent of cases are females. Prevalence in late-teenage females is between 0.5 and 1.0 percent, and there has been an increase in recent decades. It occurs more often in wealthy societies, and there is an increased risk in close family members. Mood disorders are also more common in these families. This syndrome is often an occupational risk among dancers, models, and actresses.

Onset and Course

The pattern of Anorexia is quite variable. Some individuals get well after one episode, some have a pattern of relapse and getting better, and some have a downhill course. Of severe cases admitted to teaching centers, the long-term death rate is more than 10 percent.

Treatment

Self-Help. Self-help groups include the American Anorexia/Bulimia Association, National Eating Disorders Organization, and National Association of Anorexia Nervosa and Associated Disorders. There are some useful books that one can read on this subject, including Joan Jacobs Brumberg's *The Body Project*, Hilde Bruch's *The Golden Cage: The Enigma of Anorexia Nervosa*, and Raymond Lemberg's *Eating Disorder: A Reference Sourcebook*.

Professional Help. A good medical workup is required so that a physical cause is not missed. Some of these patients may be able to be treated with psychotherapy or medications on an outpatient basis. However, some patients will require inpatient care to stabilize weight and permit recovery.

Section 2: Bulimia Nervosa

When I write of hunger, I am really writing about love and the hunger for it, and warmth and the love of it and the hunger for it . . . and then the warmth and richness and fine reality of hunger satisfied . . . and it is all one.
                        Mary Frances Kennedy Fisher, *The Gastronomical Me*, 1943

What Is the Definition?

Bulimia comes from a Greek word that means "ox-like (or big) hunger" and *nervosa* means "nerves." Bulimia involves binge eating and then use of various means to prevent weight gain.

What Are the Symptoms?

Symptoms include a pattern of binge eating followed by vomiting and sometimes use of laxatives and diuretics. These activities are accompanied by shame at the loss of control and are often done in secret. There is an exaggerated fear of gaining weight, as with Anorexia Nervosa, but these persons are mostly in the *normal weight* range. There are often depressive symptoms present.

Who Is Affected?

Bulimia mostly begins in the late teen years or early adult life, and 90 percent of sufferers are female. Among teenage and young adult females, the prevalence is 1 to 3 percent. It is more common in wealthy societies and tends to run in families. Other mental illnesses found in these families are mood disorders and substance abuse and dependence.

Onset and Course

The initial binge eating may follow a period of dieting. The course may be chronic or cyclic. The vomiting can cause loss of dental enamel and severe dental problems. The parotid glands may become swollen and the menses can be irregular. Tears of the esophagus, gastric rupture, and cardiac problems may occur.

Treatment

Self-Help. For self-help groups, see the preceding section, "Anorexia Nervosa." There is also the S.M.A.R.T. Network (Self-Management and Recovery Training) (see appendix B) for "addictive behaviors" including eating disorders. A video produced by the American Psychiatric Association called *Bulimia: The Binge-Purge Obsession* includes helpful interviews with victims of this disorder. A recent memoir of someone with Bulimia is *Wasted* by Marya Hornbacher.

Professional Help. A thorough medical workup should be performed to decide if body tissue damage has occurred from the behavior. Psychiatric evaluation and treatment is often essential.

T. Allen

Chapter 12
Sleep Disorders

Sleep that knits up the ravell'd sleave of care.

William Shakespeare, *Macbeth*, 1606

The word *sleep* comes from an Old English word, *slaf*, which means "sleep." When marked changes occur during any part of the normal sleep pattern or cycle, or when one's work, social, school, or other functions are altered by tiredness from disturbed sleep, then one has a sleep disorder. There may be a Primary Sleep Disorder or a sleep disorder caused by a mental illness, substance abuse, or a general medical illness. Among mental illnesses, sleep problems may be seen in Major Depressive Disorder, Bipolar Disorder, Schizophrenia, or Panic Disorder. Use and/or withdrawal from drugs, alcohol, psychostimulants, caffeine, cocaine, opioids, relaxants, and sedatives may cause sleep disorders. Also physical diseases of the nervous system, skeleto-muscular system, or endocrine system; infection; coughing; or simple body pains may cause sleep problems. Sleep Disorders caused by mental illness, substance abuse, or physical illness will not be discussed further, as their symptoms are the same as seen in Primary Sleep Disorders, and their treatments focus more on the primary illness than on the sleep problem itself. The Primary Sleep Disorders are Dyssomnias and Parasomnias.

Section 1: Dyssomnias

What Is the Definition?

Dyssomnia comes from the Latin prefix *dys-*, which means "bad" or "difficult," and the Latin word *somnia*, which means "sleep." Thus, Dyssomnia relates to poor sleep. Dyssomnias fall into five major subgroups: Primary Insomnia, Primary Hypersomnia, Narcolepsy, Breathing Related Disorders, and Circadian Rhythm Disorders.

What Are the Symptoms?

People who do not sleep enough have Primary *Insomnia*. People who sleep *too much* have Primary *Hypersomnia*. Those unable to resist falling asleep suddenly for a few minutes during the day have *Narcolepsy*. Those who have reduced or no breathing for many seconds during sleep (apnea) have a *Breathing-Related Disorder*. And those who have problems sleeping because of changes in work hours, airplane jet lag, or an inner delayed sleep phase have *Circadian Rhythm Disorder*.

Who Is Affected?

Below is a chart of prevalence of Sleep Disorders in the general population.

Disorder	Prevalence

Primary Insomnia
  General adults
  Elderly adults
	Up to 10%
	Up to 25%

Primary Hypersomnia General adults	Unknown
Narcolepsy	Up to 0.16%
Obstructive Breathing-Related Disorders General adults	Up to 10.0%

Circadian Rhythm Disorder
  Delayed Sleep Phase
  Night Shift Work
	Up to 7% of adolescents
	Up to 60%

Obstructive Sleep Apnea occurs mostly in middle-aged, overweight males and in children with large tonsils. It is seen up to four times more often in adult males than adult females. Similarly, central sleep apnea occurs more in males than females. The likelihood of both obstructive and central sleep apnea increases with age.

In Circadian Rhythm Disorder, the *Delayed Sleep Phase* Type occurs mostly between late childhood and early adulthood. With people in their middle or late years, one sees Shift Work Type and Jet Lag Type symptoms.

Onset and Course

Primary Insomnia may be triggered by a stress and continue after the stress resolves. Primary Hypersomnia has an onset between ages fifteen and thirty and sometimes occurs in families. Narcolepsy begins in the teen years, and up to 40 percent of such patients have another mental illness at the same time. Breathing-Related Disorders have at least three distinct causes and lower the oxygen level in the blood, sometimes causing death. Circadian Rhythm Disorders are seen in middle-age and older people who have problems with airplane jet lag or shift work changes. About 7 percent of teenagers have a delayed sleep phase that results in their being "late to bed, late to rise" which may have a cultural aspect.

Young adults with Primary Insomnia have problems *falling* asleep, while older adults have problems *staying* asleep and waking up too early. Excess use and abuse of sleeping pills are a danger. Primary Hypersomnia tends to become chronic, and excess use and abuse of stimulants are a risk. Narcolepsy causes danger when patients drive cars or use machinery. People with a Breathing Related Disorder are very tired much of the time; their sleep is broken because they often awaken gasping for air; snoring and being overweight are frequently associated. People with Circadian Rhythm Disorder are also sleepy much of the time.

Treatment

Self-Help. Books or pamphlets from the American Sleep Disorders Association can help in learning about a sleeping problem. Likewise, the book *No More Sleepless Nights*, by Peter Hauri and Shirley Linde, might also be helpful. Depending on the type of sleeping problem involved, it is possible to learn ways to change one's sleeping habits so as to bring on and maintain a restful sleep and to better control one's sleeping patterns.

Professional Help. A physician can discern if any general medical illness, mental illness, or substance abuse is causing the sleep problems and arrange for it to be treated. Sleep clinics focus on diagnosing and treating patients with sleep problems. Surgical treatment or certain breathing machines and exercises can also help relieve these symptoms. Carefully monitored medication and different presleep relaxation, yoga, meditation, and other similar techniques may help bring on and maintain sleep or affect more wakefulness as needed.

Section 2: Parasomnias

What Is the Definition?

Parasomnia is from the Latin prefix *para-*, which means "alongside of," and the Latin word *somnia*, which means "sleep." Persons with Parasomnia and their parents may complain of certain strange actions during sleep that disturb the normal sleep cycle. Parasomnias include three main subgroups: Nightmare Disorders, Sleep Terror Disorders, and Sleepwalking Disorders.

What Are the Symptoms?

Nightmares are very frightening dreams that cause sleepers to wake up suddenly in the early morning hours. On waking, they have a fast pulse and heavy breathing and are sweating. When these nightmares affect social, work, school, or personal function, one has a Nightmare Disorder. Victims of Sleep Terror Disorders sit up suddenly in terror with a loud scream or cry during the evening and nighttime hours, soon after going to sleep. They also have a rapid pulse, fast breathing, increased muscle tone, and a confused look. They cannot become fully awake nor be given comfort or relief. After a few minutes, they return rather quickly to sleep and do not recall the nighttime events the next day.

Persons with Sleepwalking Disorder carry out complex motor acts while sleeping. Such people may sit up in bed, get out of bed, move about the house, do certain tasks, and return to bed, all while still asleep. Their faces have a blank stare. They do not respond to others and recall very little of what happened the next morning.

Who Is Affected?

Nightmares may be understood in different ways depending on one's culture. One group might attribute nightmares to certain "spirits" or within a spiritual context; others might see nightmares as revealing some physical or mental illness. In fact, Nightmare Disorders often follow major stresses at home, in school, or at work. More females report nightmares than males. Conversely, more male children than female children report sleep terrors; in adults however, males and females report sleep night terrors with about the same frequency. People who have a close relative with Sleep Terror Disorder are ten times more likely than others to get the illness. In Sleepwalking Disorder, adult males may act violently, while women sometimes eat food. Girls sleepwalk more than boys, but in adults, the ratio is about even. Like Sleep Terror Disorder, Sleepwalking Disorder also runs in families. If both parents were sleepwalkers, there is a 60 percent chance their children will do likewise.

Onset and Course

Each of these subgroups has a different set of causes, age of onset, and course of illness.

Nightmares begin between ages three and six and occur in up to 50 percent of children three to five years old, but lessen over time. Females have up to four times more nightmares than males. Real-life stresses can set off nightmares. Beginning at age four through twelve, 6 percent of children have sleep terror episodes. In adults, sleep terrors develop between twenty and thirty years of age and occur less than 1 percent of the time. Sleepwalking begins between four and eight years of age, peaks among twelve-year-olds, and mostly disappears by fifteen. It rarely appears for the first time in an adult. Up to 30 percent of children have at least one sleepwalking event each year; the figure is up to 7 percent among adults. Eighty percent of sleepwalkers have a family history.

People with nightmares are often anxious and depressed. Nightmares disturb sleep, causing tiredness the next day and poor performance in school or at work. In contrast, children with sleep terrors do not fully awake, nor are they aware the next day of what occurred the night before, though adults can also cause damage to others. People with sleep terrors have other mental illnesses. Sleepwalkers can injure themselves by falling down stairs or out of windows, walking into objects, and even by going out into the street and being hurt. This illness can be brought on by fevers, sleep deprivation, sleep apnea, substance use, and neurological illnesses.

Treatment

Self-Help. Books and pamphlets may help clarify that the person has a sleep problem and may help the person seek proper health care. Self-help groups can also be useful. The National Sleep Foundation provides educational guides for persons with sleep disorders. *The Promise of Sleep: A Pioneer in Sleep Medicine Explains the Vital Connection between Health, Happiness and a Good Sleep* by William Dement, M.D., a pioneer in sleep studies, can be useful.

Professional Help. An expert can best discern whether the sleep problem is primary or due to substance use, a medical illness, or another mental illness. They may also help set up a treatment plan involving adjustments in sleep routine, sleep medication, or psychotherapy.

M. Liebman

Chapter 13
Impulse-Control Disorders

The word *impulse* comes from the Latin *impellere*, meaning "to impel" or "to drive." People with Impulse-Control Disorders feel driven to performs acts that are harmful to themselves or to others. A sense of tension before the impulsive act often leads to relief or pleasure after the act is over. There may also be regret and guilt later. There are five major Impulse-Control Disorders.

Many people can have trouble with impulse control, but minor or rare impulsive acts are not considered a disorder. People with other mental disorders can also have problems with impulse control, but a diagnosis of the disorders discussed in this chapter is made only when the acts are not part of another mental condition.

Section 1: Intermittent Explosive Disorder

To whom can I speak today?
Gentleness has perished
And the violent man has come down on everyone.
Anonymous, The Man Who Was Tired of Life, ca. 1990 B.C.

What Is the Definition?

The word *explosive* comes from the Latin *explodere*, meaning "to drive out with a violent noise." A person with Intermittent Explosive Disorder has a pattern of sudden acts during which he or she is driven by violent urges to assault or verbally threaten someone or to destroy property. These acts are much more severe than could be justified on the basis of any offense by the other person.

What Are the Symptoms?

A person with Intermittent Explosive Disorder will tend to have sudden rages at times when he or she feels stressed. There may be physical symptoms before the outbursts, such as palpitations and tightness in the chest. After an episode of rage, there may be feelings of tiredness and depression. Between such acts, this same person may show no sign of a problem, although some do show a frequently impulsive or hostile way of thinking. "Road rage" may sometimes belong under this heading.

Who Is Affected?

Intermittent Explosive Disorder is thought to be rare. It occurs more often in males than in females. In as many as 50 percent of people with this disorder, there are vague findings in neurological, brainwave, or psychological tests. There may be a record of head injury or seizures during fevers in childhood. It is not understood as yet how such findings might be related to the violent urges or the poor control of them.

Onset and Course

The onset of Intermittent Explosive Disorder can occur from childhood into the twenties, and the first observed act may occur without any warning.

Little is known about the disorder's long-term course, but it may be that as a person reaches the fifties and older, these acts are less likely to occur. Explosive episodes can occur on a regular basis over many years or may occur only infrequently. As a result of the acts, people can lose jobs and friends, be divorced, have accidents, and receive injuries and jail terms.

Treatment

Self-Help. Violence is of increasing concern in our country and worldwide. There are many resources for helping people manage violent feelings, although Intermittent Explosive Disorder itself is so infrequent that there are no major organizations and few readings directed to helping with this specific type of problem. Because of the recent violent tragedies in schools, there are accelerating efforts to develop methods for identifying and helping children and adolescents who have problems with anger and a potential for violence. Advocacy and support organizations include the Center for the Prevention of School Violence, the National Center for Injury Prevention and Control, the American Association of School Administrators, the American School Counselor Association, the National Education Association, and the National PTA. Many schools are developing successful programs for conflict resolution, emotional literacy, and peer counseling.

Professional Help. A person with this disorder is likely to be required by others to seek help. If the individual is violent, hospital treatment may be required. Careful study of the person's stress level, temperament, neurological symptoms, life events, and family and social life is important. Sometimes medications can help. Psychological education may help the person learn that the acts are not rational but rather are a sign of a disorder and need to be controlled.

Section 2: Kleptomania

Adam was but human—this explains it all. He did not want the apple for the apple's sake, he wanted it only because it was forbidden.

Mark Twain, Pudd'nhead Wilson, 1894

What Is the Definition?

Klepto- comes from the Greek *kleptein*, meaning "to steal," and *mania* comes from the Greek word meaning "madness." Kleptomania is a "stealing madness." The person with Kleptomania fails to resist the impulse to steal items that have no real use or value for him or her.

What Are the Symptoms?

Stolen items typically have little cash value, such as inexpensive pens, jewelry, or watches. Even wealthy people have been arrested for shoplifting cheap items. Most of the time, the thefts are not planned, and often there is not much effort to avoid being caught. Immediately after the act, there is pleasure or relief. Because persons with Kleptomania know that the acts are wrong and seem senseless, they may feel depressed and guilty later and may then fear being arrested.

Who Is Affected?

Kleptomania is quite rare and seems to be the case in less than 5 percent of detained shoplifters, most of them being females. The cause for the senseless acts of stealing is not known. It has been suggested that these acts are those of a child stealing as a substitute for love or to punish others by hurting themselves. There may be a childhood history of problems in the family.

Onset and Course

Acts of stealing may begin anywhere from childhood to adulthood. In one study the highest rate of stealing was twenty-seven times a month. People with Kleptomania may also have Mood Disorders, especially Major Depressive Disorder, as well as Anxiety Disorders and Eating Disorders. They may also have a pattern of compulsive buying.

Little is known about the course of Kleptomania. Three patterns have been described: brief episodes followed by long periods without such acts; long and intense periods of stealing; and courses without a clear pattern. Despite many arrests, the acts may persist, leading to heavy legal expenses, financial ruin, family breakup, and career damage.

Treatment

Self-Help. Kleptomania is not well understood. It is likely that people keep their problem secret, without anyone to talk to about it. Kleptomania has some similarities to addictions in that there is a compulsion and pleasure in the act of stealing. People are most likely to be motivated to seek help right after they are caught stealing and the behavior is revealed to family and friends. Family insistence on some kind of counseling, if combined with emotional support, can be very helpful. Supportive organizations include Shoplifters Alternative and the National Curriculum and Training Institute.

Professional Help. People with this disorder are likely to get treatment only when required to by legal or other authority. Because there may be underlying mood disorders or other mental conditions, treatment of those conditions may help end the tension-reducing acts of stealing. The person is likely to benefit from the supportive empathy of an expert who helps him or her to understand and put into perspective a troubled childhood and personal life.

Section 3: Pyromania

Tyger! Tyger! burning bright
In the forests of the night.

William Blake, "The Tyger," 1794

What Is the Definition?

Pyro- comes from the Greek for "fire," and *mania* comes from the Greek of the same word, meaning "madness." Pyromania is a "fire-setting madness." The basic feature of Pyromania is repeated acts of deliberate fire-setting. The person is excited with the thrill of fires and does not set them for profit, or because of anger, or for any specific purpose other than the urge to commit the act.

What Are the Symptoms?

Persons with Pyromania report tension or a sense of stimulation before starting fires. Because of their high interest in the topic of fire, they tend to watch fires, set off false alarms, and visit the firehouse, and may even become firefighters. They may plan in a careful manner before starting a fire, yet not care at all about harm to others or damage to property, and they may even enjoy such damage.

Who Is Affected?

The frequency of Pyromania is unknown but it seems to be rare. It occurs much more often in males than in females, and more often in people who have had learning problems, Attention-Deficit Disorder, or poor social skills. It can also be associated with alcohol problems.

Onset and Course

Acts of fire-setting can be carried out by children and teens, with more than 40 percent of those arrested being under eighteen years old. However, the specific diagnosis of Pyromania can be made only rarely in these cases.

Because it is seen rarely, the usual course of Pyromania is not known. In fact, it is not known yet what the tie might be between fire-setting in childhood and in adulthood. It seems that people tend to set fires infrequently and may stop for long periods, but the long-term course is unknown. There are significant risks to this behavior, including criminal prosecution and incarceration, serious property damage, and deaths of firefighters and citizens.

Treatment

Self-Help. Because Pyromania is diagnosed only when there is fascination and excitement in fire-setting, the person is likely to be motivated for help only when he or she has been caught. The United States Fire Administration has compiled a great deal of information about the characteristics of people who set fires, which can provide useful advice for determining whether fire-setting is based on Pyromania or other motivations and what rehabilitative resources are available.

Professional Help. It is likely that most persons seeking help are forced to do so. With treatment, the great majority of children stop setting fires. Typical response of adults to expert help is not known, but it has been suggested that 70 percent or more cease fire-setting.

Section 4: Pathological Gambling

But I do guess mos peoples gonna lose.
John Berryman, *77 Dream Songs*, "Poem No. 1," 1964

What Is the Definition?

Patho comes from the Greek *pathos*, meaning "suffering." *Gamble* comes from the Old English *gamen*, meaning "fun." The basic feature of Pathological Gambling is habitual gambling acts that may start out as enjoyable but end up in suffering, playing havoc with one's personal, family, and work life. This urge to gamble is an addiction, in that the person acts from feelings rather than with the mental discipline and careful thought of a professional gambler. As a result, whereas the latter may often win, pathological gamblers invariably lose over time.

What Are the Symptoms?

Persons who have a Pathological Gambling disorder dwell almost all the time on gambling. Gambling tends to put them in an energized, excited state. They may lie about their gambling and may begin to steal as their losses increase. When trying to avoid gambling, they may become restless and moody.

Who Is Affected?

Pathological Gambling occurs in 1 to 3 percent of adults. Its frequency is increased in areas where gambling is more easily available. Pathological gambling and alcohol problems are more common in the parents of these persons. About one in three compulsive gamblers are females, who are more likely than males to be depressed and to gamble for relief.

Onset and Course

Pathological Gambling most often begins in the early teens in males but later in females. In most cases, there are several years of recreational gambling with more and more risk-taking over time. Pathological gamblers are often competitive, seek stimulation, and become bored when times are calm, and they may have shown signs of restlessness as children. They may be workaholics with an exaggerated need for approval. The urge to gamble often increases when under stress. They may develop medical problems linked to stress, such as high blood pressure and migraine headaches. There seems to be a high frequency of Major Depressive Disorder, and such persons may gamble as a way to relieve painful feelings.

The person may gamble on a regular basis or only at times, but either way, the course is most often chronic, even though the person has often made multiple attempts to reduce or stop gambling behaviors. It is thought that Pathological Gambling is an addiction akin to alcoholism and that the courses of both conditions are similar, with risks of job loss, divorce, pauperization, unpaid debts, and even suicide. Teenage internet gambling is now becoming a serious problem.

Treatment

Self-Help. Gamblers Anonymous, Gam-Anon (for families and spouses), and Gam-a-Teen (for teenage children of gamblers) are available, and they are run much like Alcoholics Anonymous. Dropout rates can be high. The National Collegiate Athletic Association (NCAA) and Harvard Medical School Division on Addictions can provide information and advice about problems of student gambling. A video, *Compulsive Gambling: The Invisible Disease*, is available from the American Psychiatric Association.

Professional Help. When gamblers seek expert help, they are often very depressed. Twenty percent of pathological gamblers who seek treatment report having made suicide attempts. Psychological support, treatment of depression, and assistance in learning to understand the nature of their illness can be very helpful to those who stay in treatment. Hospitalization is sometimes required. As with alcoholism, it can be hard to keep the person motivated for abstinence. Long-term results of treatment efforts are likely to be about the same as for the treatment of alcoholism.

Section 5: Trichotillomania

I dream of Jeanie with the light brown hair,
Floating, like a vapor, on the soft summer air.
            Stephen Collins Foster, "Jeanie with the Light Brown Hair," 1854

What Is the Definition?

Trichotillo- comes from the Greek, meaning "hair pulling," and *mania* comes from the Greek word for "madness." Trichotillomania is "hair-pulling madness." Trichotillomania involves repeated, compulsive pulling out of one's hair, to the extent that hair loss can be seen by others. The person feels tense before pulling out hair, especially when trying to resist the impulse, with a feeling of relief or even pleasure when the hair-pulling begins.

What Are the Symptoms?

Hair-pulling may occur on any part of the body but happens most often on the head, eyebrows, and eyelashes. People with Trichotillomania may try to conceal visible signs of hair loss and deny causing it. Episodes of hair-pulling may range from brief and irregular bouts to periods that last for many hours. Hair-pulling can increase with stress but can also occur when a person seems to be relaxed. People most often engage in hair-pulling when not being observed by others. There may be a preoccupation with looking at hairs that are pulled out, along with Trichophagia, that is, eating hair. Trichophagia may lead to hair balls, which can cause pain, vomiting, bleeding, and obstruction of the intestines. Some people feel the urge to pull hairs from other people, pets, and clothes such as sweaters. Nail biting and skin scratching may also occur.

Who Is Affected?

In children, hair-pulling occurs equally in females and males, but in adults it seems to be much more frequent among females. The disorder occurs in as many as 1 to 2 percent of the population. These individuals frequently have other disorders such as mood, anxiety, eating, and substance abuse disorders.

Onset and Course

Hair-pulling most often begins in childhood or the early teens. In children, bouts may be rather common, often occurring in the setting of family or other kinds of stress, and the behavior may clear up on its own, so the diagnosis of Trichotillomania is not made unless the hair-pulling lasts for many months.

Whereas hair-pulling often clears up in childhood, this habit can be chronic in adults, often involving diverse body areas. The behavior can come and go or can be continuous for many years. Risks include embarrassed social isolation, need for hairpieces or other modes of concealment, and even plastic surgery.

Treatment

Self-Help. There are a number of books about Trichotillomania, such as *Trichotillomania: A Guide* by James Jefferson and John Greist, as well as Internet sites and chatrooms, such as the Trichotillomania Mailing List and "Go Ask Alice," produced by Columbia University. This disorder has characteristics of an Obsessive-Compulsive Disorder and information about it can be found through the Obsessive-Compulsive Foundation.

Professional Help. In the case of children, the pediatrician may look for signs of stress in the family and offer helpful suggestions that result in a better home setting, which may put an end to the hair-pulling. Psychotherapy may also be helpful for Trichotillomania. Most often, with proper professional treatment of the other disorders present, such as Mood and Anxiety Disorders, the hair-pulling stops or occurs much less often.

L. Park

Chapter 14
Adjustment Disorders

From winter, plague and pestilence, good Lord, deliver us!

Thomas Nashe, *Summer's Last Will and Testament*, 1600

What Is the Definition?

The word *adjustment* comes from the Latin *adiuxtare*, meaning "to put close to." A person with an Adjustment Disorder has symptoms that are "close to," that is, triggered by, specific events. To be certain that the symptoms are actually a reaction to these events or "stressors," the symptoms must start within three months after the stressor begins and disappear within six months after the stressor ends. The stressor must either trigger strong distress that is greater than one would normally expect or result in obvious harm to one's social or working patterns. This disorder fits into what is called a "residual" category, because the diagnosis is only made if the symptoms do not fit another disorder. Response to death of a loved one is not included ("Bereavement"—see chapter 16).

What Are the Symptoms?

There are five types of Adjustment Disorder grouped on the basis of predominant types of symptoms or behaviors: Adjustment Disorder With Depressed Mood, With Anxiety, With Mixed Anxiety and Depressed Mood, With Disturbance of Conduct, and With Mixed Disturbance of Emotions and Conduct. Disturbance of Conduct refers to acts such as reckless driving, fighting, damaging property, and refusing legal duties. There can be one or more stressors, such as loss of a job, separation and divorce, natural disaster, end of a romance, illness, retirement, and severe money crisis from stock market or other investment losses.

Who Is Affected?

The rate of occurrence of this disorder in the general population has not been determined, but it appears to be rather high. In a general hospital survey, it was found in 5 percent of patients admitted, and it is seen in 10 to 30 percent of patients in mental health offices and clinics. In the case of children and adolescents, Adjustment Disorder is seen in equal numbers of boys and girls, but in adults, it is seen twice as often in females.

Onset and Course

The onset of Adjustment Disorder tends to be rapid and with acute symptoms. Friends and others may notice a change in the person's mood as well as his or her work or study habits. Most often, an Adjustment Disorder is not long-lasting, since by definition, it must last no more than six months after the stressor is over. There can be a risk of substance abuse or even suicide. When additional symptoms occur as a result of a health problem, they may hinder recovery. There are many cases in which the stressor goes on for a long period of time, such as losing a job and being unemployed, chronic illness, or severe and lasting marital conflict. In such situations, symptoms may progress to another, more serious disorder, such as severe depression. Certain stressors can occur on a regular basis, such as for farmers living in climates with frequent floods or droughts. With natural disasters or group events, such as school shootings, a number of persons may have acute stress, but if severe symptoms are still present six months after the event has passed, then the condition may well be Posttraumatic Stress Disorder or Major Depressive Disorder (see chapters 5 and 6).

Treatment

Self-Help. Persons with Adjustment Disorders can help themselves by reaching out to their friends. If they are loners or feel they cannot talk about the symptoms or the stressor, their symptoms are likely to continue. If the person is part of a group of people hurt by the stressor, support and comfort may be available from many agencies, including the Emergency Services and Disaster Relief Branch of the Center for Mental Health Services (CMHS), the National Organization for Victim Assistance, Red Cross Disaster Services, and local social agencies and religious support groups, as well as hot lines such as Project Pave, which offers counseling for adolescent victims of violence. See appendix B for recommended books.

Professional Help. Persons with this disorder can be helped greatly when they seek professional treatment from an expert. They almost always respond well to support and to help in understanding more clearly what happened and what they can do about it. In some cases, there may be intense, inappropriate feelings of responsibility and guilt regarding serious injuries and deaths, especially in situations such as natural disasters and shootings. These feelings require very attentive support, comforting, and monitoring. Medications may be prescribed if severe symptoms do not begin to clear up fairly promptly. Even persons who have been burdened with chronic stressors can usually be helped.

L. Park

Chapter 15
Personality Disorders

The root word of personality in Latin, *persona*, refers to a mask, used in ancient times by an actor to reveal a vital aspect of a story figure. It was the emblem of the character, how they were known to the audience. This chapter describes a series of such "masks," or perceived patterns, which are known to lead to impaired bonding with others. Because human beings live in a social world, such breakdowns can have a very harmful impact on love and work, and hence they are called disorders. Though it is only an aspect of the "self," it is not always easy for people to see that. The traits are not "put on," as an actor puts on a mask, but acquired over years from experiences and perhaps some inborn aspects of temperament. It is usually in place by the late teens or early adult life.

Section 1: Paranoid Personality Disorder

For somehow this is tyranny's disease, to trust no friends.
Aeschylus, *Prometheus Bound*, 4th century B.C.

What Is the Definition?

The Greek source of the word *paranoid* ("distracted") is not very helpful, but the word has come to mean an intense distrust and suspiciousness of the motives of others.

What Are the Symptoms?

The sense of mistrust in a paranoid person is very deep and is not altered by kindness or love. Those with the disorder suspect the intent of others even in the most benign cases and may become fearful or angry, or both. If anger linked to the mistrust is strong, then the person may be cold, bear grudges, blame others, be hostile, argue, try to control others, or engage in fights or legal disputes. If fear linked to the mistrust is strong, then the person may be guarded, secret, devious, or aloof.

Who Is Affected?

Paranoid disorders are found more often in males than in females and may first be recognized in childhood among children who don't mix well with others, achieve poorly in school, are teased, or have odd or strange ideas. Paranoid Personality Disorder occurs in 0.5 to 2.5 percent of the population. There is some greater risk in persons who have a family member with Schizophrenia or Delusional Disorder.

Onset and Course

The onset of Paranoid Personality Disorder most often occurs in the teen years. Brief psychoses may occur. Both Psychotic and Major Depressive Disorders are more likely to develop, as are other mental illnesses. Work and friendships are often disrupted, and violence may occur.

Treatment

Self-Help. These traits can be adaptive in unsafe circumstances, for example, people caught in the Nazi genocide, Stalin's Purge, or the Cambodian "killing fields"; but they impair the forming of the close ties needed for normal life. Being aware of the pattern can help one to control it. A fictional character with many of these traits is Captain Queeg in Herman Wouk's *The Caine Mutiny.*

Professional Help. The need for and extent of expert help will vary with the degree of impairment and other disorders. With psychosis or Major Depressive Disorder, inpatient care may be required. With impaired self-care, day hospital treatment may be needed. Outpatient psychotherapy and/or medication may be useful for milder forms.

T. Allen

Section 2: Schizoid Personality Disorder

O what can ail thee, knight-at-arms,
Alone and palely loitering?
The sedge has withered from the lake,
And no birds sing!

John Keats, *La Belle Dame sans Merci,* 1820

What Is the Definition?

Schizoid comes from the Greek *schiz-*, meaning "separated," and *-oid*, meaning "like"—so, "like separated." The central feature of Schizoid Personality Disorder is a detachment from others and from one's own feelings.

What Are the Symptoms?

People with Schizoid Personality Disorder are "loners," don't respond aptly to social cues, show only a narrow range of feelings, and often pursue tasks and hobbies that have few or no social aspects to them. There is a reduced sense of pleasure— social, emotional, or sexual. They have trouble with feeling anger and appear indifferent to praise or reproach. In childhood, poor peer relations may be noted, as well as underachievement in school. Teasing of them is common in the teen years, because these people are seen as "odd."

Who Is Affected?

Schizoid Personality Disorder occurs slightly more often in males than females. This disorder may be found in as much as 7 percent of the population at large. The pattern is present by the time of young adulthood. Their families may have an increased likelihood of Schizophrenia or Schizotypal Personality Disorder.

Onset and Course

Persons with this disorder under stress may have brief episodes of psychosis or may develop a chronic form of a psychotic disorder. Their lives may lack purpose or aim, they often do not marry, and they work best in isolated settings.

Treatment

Self-Help. Social contact may be stressful for those with Schizoid Personality Disorder, but it is often protective against psychotic events. However, the person does need to be able to withdraw from others to protect himself or herself from overly intense feelings.

Professional Help. Psychotic episodes may require hospital care, but psychotherapy with medication to help manage painful feelings about stressful events can assist the patient to live a useful and productive life.

T. Allen

Section 3: Schizotypal Personality Disorder

Those whom God wishes to destroy,
He first makes mad.

Euripides, ca. 455–406 B.C.

What Is the Definition?

The root words here do not set this diagnosis apart from the prior one. What is common among the two disorders is the detachment from others, but what is distinct here is the strange thoughts and ideas.

What Are the Symptoms?

The strange ideas associated with Schizotypal Personality Disorder may include thoughts that the affected persons has a sixth sense so that they know future events, that outside events have a special meaning for them, that they can read others' thoughts, or that they have "magical" control over others. Their speech may be vague, or "loose," or may contain odd turns of phrase. Their dress may be unkempt or bizarre; they may avoid eye contact, and are often thought eccentric. They may also mistrust and be suspicious of others.

Who Is Affected?

About 3 percent of the population is affected, and it is slightly more common in males than females. There may be a family background of Schizophrenia. Poor peer relations and underachievement in school during childhood often precede it. Teasing by others because of being odd is common in the teen years.

Onset and Course

Persons with Schizotypal Personality Disorder may have anxiety or depressive symptoms and may also have brief psychoses. Some may endure more long-term psychotic symptoms. More than half have at least one bout of Major Depressive Disorder.

Treatment

The self-help and professional treatments for Schizotypal Personality Disorder are the same as those for Schizoid Personality Disorder.

T. Allen

Section 4: Antisocial Personality Disorder

Appearances often are deceiving.
Aesop, "The Wolf in Sheep's Clothing," ca. 550 B.C.

What Is the Definition?

The term *anti-* comes from the Greek for "opposite," and the word *social* comes from the Latin word *socius*, meaning "companion." People with Antisocial Personality Disorder have patterns of actions toward others that are the opposite of those one expects from a friend or companion, that is, they don't care about and trespass on the rights of others.

What Are the Symptoms?

Because people with Antisocial Personality Disorder do not respect the rights of others, they may break laws and are often arrested and jailed. They tend to lie and deceive for their own gain and may lack concern for the safety of themselves and others. They can easily be hostile and may have a history of repeated fights or attacks on people. They can also be quite impulsive—for instance, quitting a job on the spur of the moment because of dislike for something minor—and in general they are highly irresponsible, not keeping promises, not paying debts, or not being at all faithful when married. Although people with this disorder may have good verbal talents and may put on a show of being sorry about their acts, they most often do not care and lack empathy about what happens to others whom they have abused. However, they can often take on the *role* of a sincere, honest, engaging, or reformed person, and that is why they have the reputation of being good at "conning"others.

Who Is Affected?

About 2 percent of the population has this condition, with three out of four of those being males. Close relatives are more likely to have the disorder and to have drug or alcohol problems.

Onset and Course

Children who are going to develop Antisocial Personality Disorder show signs of Conduct Disorder (see Disruptive Behavior Disorders in chapter 1) by the early teens. They may have a history of child abuse or neglect, or erratic household rules and discipline.

Sadly, these people seem to sabotage themselves over and over, often ending up with severe legal problems or in jail, and they do not learn from experience. Although the personality type persists through adult life, the behaviors tend to decrease or even stop as the person gets beyond the thirties or forties. Sometimes it is said that the urges fueling their actions "burn out" with age. They may also develop other disorders, such as depression, substance abuse, and impulse control disorders. Their life spans may be shorter because they are more likely than others to die at a young age from violent events, including homicide and suicide.

Treatment

Self-Help. If people with Antisocial Personality Disorder can gain a sense that they are wasting their lives, there are many social agencies available for them, as well as many books and other written materials.

Professional Help. Persons with this disorder do not seek expert help for this disorder itself. They may seek help because they feel defeated and depressed or because they are very anxious about something, but they seem unable to really grasp the idea of trying to change the way they think about themselves and others. In addition to seeking help for symptoms of distress, they may see experts because they are required to do so by the legal system or because they want to convince someone that they really plan to reform, for instance, a spouse who wants a divorce. Only in milder cases is there evidence that treatment can succeed beyond mere symptom relief.

L. Park

Section 5: Borderline Personality Disorder

I hate and I love. Why I do so, perhaps you ask.
    I know not, but I feel it and I am in torment.

Gaius Valerius Catallus, *Carmina*, c. 54 B.C.

What Is the Definition?

Borderline means "on the border" or "on the edge." This word was first used to describe an illness with symptoms so severe and dramatic that such patients were thought to be quite close to or "on the border of" Schizophrenia. It has become clear, however, that they are neither close to nor do they become schizophrenic.

What Are the Symptoms?

Borderline Personality Disorder (BPD) is a severe, life-threatening illness that pervades most aspects of living, such as bonds to others, sense of self, mood, and conduct. Affected people tend to feel almost constant psychic pain, weighed down by self-hate and by intense, painful relationships, with longing for closeness and yet fear of trusting others, and they may make frantic efforts to avoid feared loss of the other. They often act on impulse, with results that may be harmful to them. They feel empty and depressed, sometimes with sudden cycles of severe depression and suicide attempts, and they may injure themselves as a way to reduce the psychic pain. They are often very unsure about who they are, what they value, and what they want in life. They can quickly become confused and enraged in stressful contacts with others, which can briefly progress to paranoid ideas and symptoms of dissociation (see chapter 9). At other times, they can be quite winsome, responsive to the needs of others, and even put up with abusive people.

Who Is Affected?

About 2 percent of the population has this disorder, with three out of four of those being females. Childhood histories most often reveal marked physical, sexual, and/or psychological abuse of these individuals who were often sensitive and even pliant as small children.

Onset and Course

Borderline Personality Disorder appears by the teen or early adult years. Since teens often have problems with sense of self and with relationships, care must be taken in making this diagnosis before adulthood.

Ten percent of borderline persons commit suicide, most often in the early years of their illness. In one major study, it was found that more than a third of women who had Borderline Personality Disorder along with marked depression and alcohol abuse committed suicide.

Many people have thought of those with this disorder as unreliable and not helped by treatment, making suicide threats and causing other crises, but follow-up studies have shown that over time with treatment, the great majority of them improve. By fifteen years after initial diagnosis, two-thirds of surviving patients are no longer borderline and are functioning normally or with only minimal symptoms.

Treatment

Self-Help. Persons with Borderline Personality Disorder often look for self-help resources, which are found in bookstores and on the Internet. They can be helped greatly by finding friends who can endure their distrust and sudden changes in mood. It is known that most people do recover, and also that they are often found, sometimes not until later, to be sensitive, intuitive, and creative. For books and other references, see appendix B.

Professional Help. People with this disorder often require both psychotherapy and medications from experts who are skilled in treating them. Skillful psychotherapy can help them through crises, provide them with steady support that promotes the growth of trust, and relieve their sense of great confusion and self-hate by helping them learn what happened to them in their early years. Although there is no specific drug treatment for the borderline disorder itself, such treatment is usually helpful for symptoms of psychic pain and distress, the most frequent and painful of which are those of depression. Patients may also require treatment for symptoms of other disorders, such as anxiety, phobic, posttraumatic, substance abuse, eating, and panic disorders, as well as other personality disorders. Brief hospitalization may be required at times of extreme distress and suicidal intention.

L. Park

Section 6: Histrionic Personality Disorder

All the world's a stage,
And all the men and women merely players.
William Shakespeare, *As You Like It*, 1599

What Is the Definition?

Histrionic means "theatrical" or "dramatic." This term replaced *hysterical* (root word *hystera*, meaning "of the womb" in Greek), which was felt to incorrectly convey that it was mainly a disorder of females.

What Are the Symptoms?

Histrionic Personality Disorder describes someone who tends to use styles often employed "on stage," but which are viewed as false away from that setting. "Showy" dress, "stage" responses, speech lacking detail, constant flirting, "fishing for compliments," and always seeking the spotlight in social settings are some of the traits. The person may feel people known only briefly, or not well, to be closer friends than they really are, showering them with physical affection and trusting them too much. There is also a penchant to engage in romantic fancy. An impaired bond with members of the same sex is common. The affected person may realize that he or she is overly "clingy" but find it hard to resist the need to have others agree or approve.

Who Is Affected?

The portrait of this disorder goes back to the time of the Greeks. It is found in all cultures, in both sexes, and in about 2 to 3 percent of the overall population. Temperament plays a role, but so do other factors. For instance, anger at not being the center of attention may mask intense fears of being rejected. Exaggerated emotion may mask fear of not being taken seriously. Not giving precise dates or details may be a style used to avoid thinking about painful events.

Onset and Course

Histrionic Personality Disorder appears first in the teen years or early twenties. These individuals may seek help in dealing with a failed romance or marriage. The failure often results from the trouble that they have with real closeness in love and with sexual feelings. Being inclined to flirt and to get "bored" may lead to affairs, which, when found out, end the union, or threaten to, which sends the patient into a panic to seek help. The patient's partner may find the constant demands for attention, or the emotional storms, too much and may seek to end the contact, with the same result. There is a higher risk of suicidal gestures in people with this disorder, and a bent toward developing physical symptoms.

Treatment

Self-Help. Having strong friendships with both sexes provides a balance and can offer support during times of crisis. One can observe a fictional character, Carmen, in Bizet's opera of the same name, with many of these traits.

Professional Help. The major approach to Histrionic Personality Disorder is psychotherapy, or psychoanalysis, where the patient can explore feelings that lie beneath the symptoms that often get him or her into trouble. It is when these feelings have been brought to conscious knowledge and are under conscious control that the patient has a real chance to avoid the results that have been so painful in the past.

Medication to help the patient through acute symptoms brought on by the breakup of a relationship may be prescribed.

T. Allen

Section 7: Narcissistic Personality Disorder

He was like a cock who thought the sun had risen to hear him crow.
George Eliot, *Adam Bede*, 1859

What Is the Definition?

The word *narcissistic* comes from Narcissus, a handsome youth of Greek myth who pined away with love for his own reflection. A person with Narcissistic Personality Disorder is obsessed with an extreme need to be admired, has a very grandiose picture of himself or herself, and at the same time lacks feelings for others.

What Are the Symptoms?

People with Narcissistic Personality Disorder have a marked sense of self-importance that is not based on the facts. They believe they are special and should be admired by others, yet their self-esteem can often be shaken temporarily. They may have frequent daydreams about their talents, abilities, and great futures. They feel worthy of special notice by other people and can become very angry if it is absent. On the other hand, if things are going their way, they can often be quite charming. They tend to exploit people for what they want because they do not care to or cannot tune in to the feelings and needs of others. They may also look down on people, and if someone has special qualities, even just being happy, they can quickly become envious. Any or all of these ways of being may be deliberately concealed so that a casual observer might see only the mask of an idealistic, driven, or highly responsible person.

Who Is Affected?

Less than 1 percent of the population has Narcissistic Personality Disorder, with apparently the majority being male. They may also have mood, eating, and substance abuse problems, as well as other personality disorders.

Onset and Course

Narcissistic Personality Disorder appears by the teens or early adult years. However, many teens who show these characteristics do not progress to the disorder as adults.

This disorder was once thought to be highly stable throughout a person's life course. However, a recent study found that there tends to be some improvement in a majority, although others don't change over time.

Treatment

Self-Help. Sometimes a person with Narcissistic Personality Disorder might have some sense that there is a problem with feeling special and may then try to learn to compensate. Many resources in literature reveal narcissistic characteristics, for example, several of Charles Dickens's characters, including Steerforth and his mother in *David Copperfield*.

Professional Help. People with this disorder believe that their ways of thinking are right, so they usually do not try to help themselves unless they become depressed or get into trouble, for instance, with legal, job-related, financial, or marital problems. If they do look to others, quite often it is to get their way or to make others change without changing themselves. They can be helped by experts who are especially trained to look for signs of this disorder. For instance, such a person may seek help for depression resulting from failure to achieve unrealistic goals or failure to succeed in controlling others. The depression may respond to a supportive therapist who can be admiring of the person's engaging ways. However, unless the expert can detect the deeper mental outlook, the person may end up in better spirits but with the same troublesome attitudes that got him or her into difficulty in the first place.

L. Park

Section 8: Avoidant Personality Disorder

And how am I to face the odds
Of Man's Bedevilment and God's?
I, a stranger and afraid
In a world I never made.

Alfred E. Housman, *Last Poems*, 1922

What Is the Definition?

The word *avoidant* comes from the Latin *a-*, which means "away from," and *void*, which means "empty." People with avoidant personalities stay away from or keep empty distance between themselves and others in a distant, cautious, frightened manner or style.

What Are the Symptoms?

People with Avoidant Personality Disorder are very fearful of not being able to achieve and not being good enough to carry out the usual tasks of life. In turn, they shrink from what they feel will be harsh judgments, critiques, and not being approved. They may be quick to hear others as critics of their ideas and interests. They are afraid of being shamed, have low self-esteem, stay away from contacts with people on a one-to-one basis, and avoid people in groups. While these people want the feeling of closeness to others, their fears of being pushed away or humiliated cause them to take a long time to trust someone. Others describe these people as being shy, timid, lonely, or quiet.

Who Is Affected?

Different cultures and ethnic groups have different standards for what constitutes being shy and retiring, or confident and outgoing. Also people from one culture who migrate or immigrate into a new culture may hesitate to speak up or pursue their rightful goals or rewards. Females may be socialized to be shy or quiet. However, this behavior as a disorder affects women and men equally. It is said to occur in up to 1 percent of the general public and makes up 10 percent of mental health outpatients.

Onset and Course

Avoidant Personality Disorder may begin with small children who are shy or fearful, and although most children outgrow such traits by their teen years, a small number continue to avoid classmates and their social group.

By adulthood, these people are clearly unsure and timid, and they quickly become hurt or offended by others. They avoid meeting new people and may avoid courting or dating; they might stay away from a job interview or react to a mundane event as if it carried great risk or danger. Thus, their work at school or at a job suffers. Such people are afraid of being seen crying or blushing. These symptoms are also seen in people with other mental illnesses, for instance, mood and anxiety disorders, Dependent Personality Disorder, or Social Phobia.

Treatment

Self-Help. People can read books about how to overcome one's fear of accepting others in a more trusting manner. Most avoidant people see their caution as necessary to protect them from showing their defects or protect them from other people. Most people with this personality disorder initially seek help because of feeling anxious or depressed. A support group for these people is Fear of Success Anonymous.

Professional Help. Therapy can help patients learn about their fears and real limits and how to change their actions so as to function better. Medicines may help relieve some of their symptoms, such as being anxious or depressed.

M. Liebman

Section 9: Dependent Personality Disorder

The night has a thousand eyes,
And the day but one;
Yet the light of the bright world dies
With the dying sun.
The mind has a thousand eyes,
And the heart but one;
Yet the light of the whole life dies
When love is done.

Francis William Bourdillon, *Among the Flowers*, 1878

What Is the Definition?

The word *dependent* comes from the Latin prefix *de-*, which means "down from," and the Latin word *pendent*, which means "hanging." Dependent people "hang onto" other people who tell them what to do, even if they are of an age to decide most things for themselves.

What Are the Symptoms?

People with Dependent Personality Disorder have a great need to be cared for and to be told what to do and how to do things. They need to be assured that their actions are correct. Those who decide for these people are most often parents, spouses, or friends. Because the patients are so passive and fearful of losing the support of those who direct them, they will often agree to do things that are not in their best interests and sometimes are harmful. They often hold in their anger and become depressed. These people are often harsh in their self-judgment and call themselves "stupid." They avoid making decisions or starting new projects until the decisions or projects are approved by their mentors.

Who Is Affected?

Culture and ethnic mores greatly affect how people learn to depend on others and how independent they become in their daily lives. Certain cultures foster being passive, helpless, and fearful, more often in females than in males. In children and adolescents, Dependent Personality Disorder may be difficult to recognize. Women may be given this diagnosis more often than men, but some studies suggest both sexes suffer equally. This disorder is seen in the general public in up to 2 to 3 percent of people.

Onset and Course

Children who have a chronic physical illness or have experienced the loss of a parent are often fearful and may become very dependent adults. They feel so bereft of any inner asset or being capable as a person that they put themselves into settings that both overprotect and sharply limit them. They don't achieve their potential as adults and feel very upset when they lose the person on whom they feel so dependent. These dependent traits are often seen in other mental disorders, such as mood and anxiety disorders, and in other personality disorders, such as Histrionic Personality and Avoidant Personality Disorders. They are also seen in people with general medical conditions.

Treatment

Self-Help. People with Dependent Personality Disorder may seek relief from others due to being depressed or anxious. Gradually they realize they are too dependent on other people. At this point, they may want to change their dependent ways and may read books about being able to decide and assert one's own thoughts about a matter. Self-help groups can offer support in these efforts. One such group is Co-Dependence Anonymous (CODA).

Professional Help. Psychotherapy on a one-to-one basis or within a group can be especially helpful if the patient wants to change his or her actions. Likewise, medications can help lower one's feelings of anxiety and depression.

M. Liebman

Section 10: Obsessive-Compulsive Personality Disorder

Faultily faultless, icily regular, spendidly null
Dead perfection, no more.

Alfred, Lord Tennyson, *Maud*, 1855

What Is the Definition?

The word *obsess* comes from the Latin word *obsidere* and means "to besiege" or "beset." In this context, to be *obsessive* means that a person is beset or besieged by thoughts that are difficult to put aside. The word *compulsion* comes from the Latin word *compellere*, which means "to compel" or "to force." Someone with this personality disorder feels compelled or forced to behave in certain ways. Obsessive-Compulsive Personality Disorder differs from Obsessive-Compulsive Disorder (see chapter 6) as the former is a whole pattern of rigid conduct, faultless to a fault, in contrast to the latter, which is made up of isolated behaviors and ideas.

What Are the Symptoms?

People with Obsessive-Compulsive Personality Disorder are obsessed with order, with being perfect, with being in control, and often with being in control of other people. Their very strict sense of right and wrong, good and bad, perfect and imperfect, control and lack of control makes handling everyday life events very difficult. They feel compelled to make detailed lists and to follow order and schedules at the cost of losing sight of the purpose of the major task to be done. As a result, they tend not to regard the welfare of others. People with such traits do not get along with or work well with other people. Jobs often do not get finished on time or even completed at all because of the patient's irrational perfectionism. Work becomes the major goal of life. There is little time for leisure. Play becomes "serious" and without purpose. These people often fit the old saying, "All work and no play makes Johnny a dull boy." They also have a problem trying to discard old, worn-out objects, which in turn may pile up and overwhelm them. They are seen as "rigid" and "right to a fault." Work, social, and other areas have sharp and severe limits. Friendships are few and life is a burden.

Who Is Affected?

Culture and ethnic groups can greatly affect how people view work, relations with others, and goal achievement. Males are diagnosed twice as often as females with this disorder. In mental health clinics, 3 to 10 percent of outpatients have this diagnosis; in the general public, about 1 percent do.

Onset and Course

The traits of being perfect, strict, and right are mostly fixed by early adulthood and are long-lasting. Cultures can breed such traits, which, in a much more limited and careful extent, can often be useful in life.

People with Obsessive-Compulsive Personality Disorder have problems getting work done and working well with others. Their strict, rigid manner can push away others. It may lead to conflicts on the job or in a marriage. These traits applied in a milder form can help one and assist in reaching goals or having a job done well.

Treatment

Self-Help. Books and self-help groups can consulted to for help in reducing these symptoms. One such group is Workaholics Anonymous World Service Organization. The book *The New Personality Self-Portrait: Why You Think, Work, Love, and Act the Way You Do*, by Lois B. Morris and John M. Oldham, can be helpful.

Professional Help. Psychotherapy on a one-to-one basis and group therapy can be helpful, as can be certain medicines in dealing with mood and anxiety disorders seen with this disorder.

M. Liebman

Chapter 16
Other Conditions

This chapter covers some disorders that do not fall well into other broader groupings. They deserve to be mentioned and described for the reader, who can then find more information on the subjects in other texts.

Section 1: Psychological Factors Affecting Medical (Physical) Conditions

Man is sometimes extraordinarily passionately in love with suffering.
Fyodor Dostoyevsky, *Notes from the Underground*, 1864

What Is the Definition?

Psyche is the Greek word for "soul" or "mind," that is, what is not of the physical world. *Physical* comes from the Greek word meaning "nature." Hence, these disorders describe ways that the mind affects the human body.

What Are the Symptoms?

The essence of this syndrome is that the onset or course of a physical illness is closely joined to clear mental or behavioral factors. This may occur through:
- *mental disorders*, for instance, the risk of dying from a heart attack is greater in persons having a Major Depressive Disorder
- *mental symptoms*, for instance, anxiety attacks can trigger asthma
- *personality traits*, for instance, having a "Type A" personality increases a person's risk of heart disease
- *harmful habits*, for instance, unsafe sex methods can lead to HIV
- *stress response*, for instance, may cause heart rhythm changes.

Who Is Affected?

The role of mental factors in the onset of a disease varies by the disorder and the patient. Just as some people respond strongly to a placebo and others do not, so one person's disease may be strongly affected by mental factors and another's not. We do not know why. Also, a medical illness itself can be a stress and induce mental symptoms.

Onset and Course

Mental factors can be as difficult to modify as physical ones, but where they are present, they have a powerful effect.

Treatment

Self-Help. Knowing the great impact that the mind can have on the health of the body gives a person a vital tool in fighting this aspect of an illness. This is not the same as saying that mental factors are the sole cause and cure, a common error. Dean Ornish in *Love and Survival: The Scientific Basis for the Healing Power of Intimacy* has outlined data showing the powerful impact of mental factors on illness and survival.

Professional Help. Someone expert in these disorders can help a patient deal with a preexisting mental ailment or stress or with the feelings that arise from having a disease. The power of this help can be seen with victims of cancer, where studies show that many patients live longer with some form of mental health treatment.

T. Allen

Section 2: Medication-Induced Movement Disorders

There are some remedies worse than the disease.
Publilius Syrus, *Maxim 301*, First Century B.C.

What Is the Definition?

Some medications, such as neuroleptics, cause muscle movements that are very hard to control. The word *neuroleptic* comes from the Greek words *neuron*, which means "nerve," and *leptiko*, which means "seize" or "take." Neuroleptics "seize" or "take" nerves, causing muscles to move in a strange, unnatural, way. These medications are prescribed for some severe mental illnesses.

What Are the Symptoms?

Medication-Induced Movement Disorders include six groups, five of which are caused by neuroleptic medicines; the sixth group is caused by other medicines also used for mental problems. The six groups are:

- Neuroleptic Parkinsonism—Mild tremors of the hands and fingers while they lie at rest, but no tremors of the hands and fingers when moving them on purpose; rigid muscles and restless movements
- Neuroleptic Malignant Syndrome—Rigid muscles, high fever, sweating, loss of bowel and bladder control, unstable blood pressure
- Neuroleptic-Induced Acute Dystonia—Muscles of the head, neck, limb, or trunk appear fixed in a certain frozen manner
- Neuroleptic-Induced Acute Akathisia—Restless body movements, fidgeting, "ants in the pants"
- Tardive Dyskinesia—Slow writhing movements, mostly about the tongue, jaw, or limb; protruding and quivering tongue; facial grimaces
- Medication-Induced Postural Tremor—A fine shaking when moving, occurring with certain nonneuroleptic drugs, such as lithium and antidepressants

Who Is Affected?

Persons who take neuroleptics or other psychoactive medicines and then get symptoms of abnormal body movements are thought to have a Medication-Induced Movement Disorder. Tardive Dyskinesia is seen more often in women.

Onset and Course

These movement problems most often begin a week or two after certain medicines that have been prescribed. Tardive Dyskinesia may come about after several years of taking a neuroleptic.

Muscles move in an arrhythmic pattern that appears strange and fitful. As a result, muscles perform their tasks poorly and awkwardly. Sometimes patients who have these movement symptoms stop taking the medicine without telling their doctor and become ill. If the medication is not reduced or stopped or other medicines are not prescribed to counter these side effects, movement symptoms will remain and worsen. In some cases, such as with Tardive Dyskinesia, the movements sometimes cannot be reversed. Neuroleptic Malignant Syndrome has caused death in some patients. These very same movements can sometimes be present in patients who have not taken any drugs; for example, some anxiety disorders can cause the same movements as those seen with Neuroleptic-Induced Acute Akathisia. Catatonia (see chapter 5) can have some of the same symptoms as Neuroleptic Malignant Syndrome. Tardive Dyskinesia was described in patients even before neuroleptics were developed.

Treatment

Self-Help. Patients who take these drugs should be informed that sometimes medication-induced movements may occur as a side effect. It is important that they call the doctor for advice before abruptly stopping the medicine on their own, which may risk a rapid return of severe symptoms.

Professional Help. A physician should assess the movements and decide which changes to make in the prescribed medication. The doctor may prescribe an additional medicine to counter the movement side effects or may have to stop the medicine altogether and prescribe a new drug for the patient's mental illness.

M. Liebman

Section 3: Other Syndromes

Other problems and stresses that can become the major focus of concern to mental health experts are briefly summarized here.

Relational Problems

The word *relational* comes from the Latin word *relatus*, meaning "brought." Relational problems involve patterns of relating among people who have been brought together into "relational units" by blood or circumstance, such as parents and children, husbands and wives, intimate partners, siblings, students, and coworkers. An example would be extreme parental overprotection that fosters withdrawn or rebellious behaviors in the children.

Bereavement

The word *bereave* comes from the Old English word *bereafian*, meaning "to take away." Bereavement is a state of extreme grief after a person who is loved has been taken away by death. Symptoms of severe depression occur, including feelings of being utterly alone and hopeless, a sense of great pain, insomnia, loss of appetite, and weight loss. If such symptoms last more than two months, then the diagnosis is changed from Bereavement to Major Depressive Disorder (see chapter 5). Early signs that it may be the latter are extreme guilt and feelings of worthlessness, severe trouble with daily life activities, intense thoughts of wishing for death, or suicidal thinking. In the case of Bereavement, strong support and guidance, and sometimes brief therapy and even medication, result in noticeable improvement within two months after the death of the loved person.

Problems Related to Abuse or Neglect

This phrase is used when the central concern of the mental health expert has to do with physical abuse, sexual abuse, or neglect. *DSM–IV–TR* provides different numerical codes that clarify when the focus of the expert is on the victim and when it is on the perpetrator (see appendix A). An example of the latter would be a parent who has given in to beating a child when angry, and who now receives expert help to learn to manage strong feelings and to provide parental guidance without resorting to violence. For victim syndromes, see also Reactive Attachment Disorder of Infancy or Early Childhood (chapter 1), and Posttraumatic Stress Disorder (chapter 6).

Malingering

The word *malinger* comes from the French word *malingre*, meaning "sickly." A person is found to be malingering when he or she either feigns illness or greatly overstates physical and mental symptoms. This is done because the person wants to avoid something, such as jail or work, or wants to obtain something, such as insurance payments or drugs.

Age-Related Cognitive Decline

The word *cognition* comes from the Latin word *cognoscere*, meaning "to learn." A normal result of aging is that one's mind does not work or learn as quickly, memory is not as good, and one may have more trouble solving problems. If a person is very troubled by such changes, yet testing shows that the changes are within the normal range for his or her age, then the focus of attention is called Age-Related Cognitive Decline. Testing and then reassurance by an expert who explains the findings to the person is almost always quite helpful.

Summary

Onset and course of symptoms, stresses, and problems in this section can vary greatly. In all cases, there are many options in the community for self-help. Several references are listed in appendix B. Most of these problems respond well to professional help, except for cases of habitual malingering or chronic abuse of others.

L. Park

Conclusions

Where Do We Go from Here?

In the introduction, we said that identifying and describing mental disorders is a work in progress (as is true with general medical disorders). The history of medicine can be seen as a few keen observers picking out the figure from the background and recognizing a pattern where others saw merely random chaos. When that pattern was found to repeat itself, it became an object of study that led to further knowledge and control, whether the control came in the form of prevention or treatment. Mental disorders are characterized by a group of signs and symptoms, i.e., syndromes, without clear known causal agents. There is therefore an element of uncertainty as to exactly where the limits of a disorder lie. But not knowing exactly where the limits lie has also made identifying causes difficult, because we cannot be sure whether researchers are studying several different disorders or the same one.

Another way of saying this is: "What *exactly* constitutes 'caseness'?" That is, what is a case of a particular disorder? There are concerns about "false positives," meaning cases labeled as of a specific disorder that are not, and "false negatives," cases not identified as of a certain type that, in fact, should be. There is also the question of whether we are splitting apart disorders that really should be lumped together or lumping together disorders that should be split apart. The powerful tools that we have acquired to study the human genome are, in the end, only as good as our accuracy in making judgments about such issues.

And mental illness is more than mental disorders. Disorders are like islands that emerge above the sea while the lesser but more common dysfunctions are like reefs and shoals upon which many lives founder. These "reefs and shoals" are not so neatly identified. In fact, there is much debate in the field about how to handle this in the writing of the next diagnostic manual of mental disorders. An example of the problem can be found in the realm of depressive symptoms. Depressive symptoms may occur in a patient, symptoms that do not rise to the level of a disorder in *DSM–IV–TR*, yet research has shown they can cause as much disability as many common medical disorders. Does that mean that our criterion are too narrow? It raises the question about how good our current maps are.

DSM–IV–TR speaks not of disease, or illness, but of disorders; therefore an important question is: What is meant by a disorder? Or to put it another way: What is disordered? This is not always answered in a consistent way. For example, in Psychosis it is the vital function of reality testing that is disordered. In Dementias, it is the vital function of memory and orientation in the world. In Mood Disorders, it is the vital function of mood regulation. In Tics and Conversion Disorders, it is the vital function of motor control. In Sleep, Eating, and Sexual Disorders, it is those vital functions. These are important basic creature tasks. On the other hand,

Personality Disorders do not represent a dysfunction at that basic level but rather in specifically human and social tasks, that is, being able to maintain and balance connections with others. Yet we are human, so dysfunction in the higher-order tasks affects those at the creature level, and vice versa. We do not understand very well the interplay at this time, but once it is worked out, it could again change how we describe mental disorders.

Another question is whether the syndrome, *or the vulnerability to it*, is the disorder. And does the syndrome create the vulnerability or does a vulnerability, given the right circumstances, lead to the syndrome? And if it is the latter, does the vulnerability only occur genetically in certain individuals, or is the vulnerability universal and a part of being human? And if the vulnerability is part of being human, is it a harmful extension of universal responses to life experiences, and adaptations to them, or due to the intricate interaction of brain development and environment that is our biological legacy (Murphy's Law: "If anything can go wrong, it will")? Do all vulnerabilities get expressed in disorders eventually, or are there some things that are protective? Are some experiences so toxic that they create vulnerability where it otherwise would not occur? Do the underlying vulnerabilities to the syndrome change over time, or do people just learn to manage them better? What is the role of meaning? Although there is no shortage of speculation and opinion, there is a serious shortage of hard data. The truth is, at this time we know little about possible underlying vulnerability issues.

Questions like these are responsible for the continuing changes in the *Diagnostic and Statistical Manual of Mental Disorders*. Each edition represents the consensus of experts as to where the science and the therapeutics are at the time it is published (every decade or so); however, one must recognize that we still have many more questions than answers. And humility is in order, for the conventional wisdom is often wrong. Patients, families, schools, and doctors would like to have more certainty, but all have to recognize that we are still a long way from that. Indeed, a work in progress!

T. Allen

How to Use the Appendix Sections

The appendixes in A *Primer of Mental Disorders* are:

Appendix A: Numerical Listing of DSM–IV–TR Diagnoses and Codes
Appendix B: Listing of Advocacy and Self-Help Resources
Appendix C: Sources of Additional Information for the Layperson for Diagnoses, Medication, Psychotherapy, Referrals
Appendix D: Mental Health Web Site Resources for Educators, Families, and Students

Appendix A is a numerical listing of all the DSM–IV diagnoses and codes. The reader should use the index to locate information about the disorder. For rarer conditions not included in the chapters, refer to the *DSM–IV–Text Revision*.

Each chapter in the *Primer* contains a self-help section that identifies key sources of information for the various topics. Appendix B includes advocacy and support organizations, survivors' accounts, as well as videos, movies, and books that pertain to the section discussed in the text. Under videos, those that are cited as produced by the American Psychiatric Association can be obtained by calling 800-366-8455 or 202-682-6349, or visit their Web site, http://www.psych.org/catalog/contents.html.

Appendix C is a listing of organizations of professionals that deal with the mental disorders listed as well as federal government agencies that may be of help.

Appendix D lists Web sites of interest to educators, families, and students with links to other resources about teaching and learning materials.

Appendix A
Numerical Listing of
DSM–IV–TR Diagnoses and Codes

To maintain compatibility with ICD-9-CM, some DSM-IV diagnoses share the same code numbers. NOS = Not Otherwise Specified. Reprinted with permission from the *Diagnostic and Statistical Manual of Mental Disorders, Fourth Edition*, © 1994 American Psychiatric Association.

290.40	Vascular Dementia, Uncomplicated
290.41	Vascular Dementia, With Delirium
290.42	Vascular Dementia, With Delusions
290.43	Vascular Dementia, With Depressed Mood
291.0	Alcohol Intoxication Delirium
291.0	Alcohol Withdrawal Delirium
291.1	Alcohol-Induced Persisting Amnestic Disorder
291.2	Alcohol-Induced Persisting Dementia
291.3	Alcohol-Induced Psychotic Disorder, With Hallucinations
291.5	Alcohol-Induced Psychotic Disorder, With Delusions
291.81	Alcohol Withdrawal
291.89	Alcohol-Induced Anxiety Disorder
291.89	Alcohol-Induced Mood Disorder
291.89	Alcohol-Induced Sexual Dysfunction
291.89	Alcohol-Induced Sleep Disorder
291.9	Alcohol-Related Disorder NOS
292.0	Amphetamine Withdrawal
292.0	Cocaine Withdrawal
292.0	Nicotine Withdrawal
292.0	Opioid Withdrawal
292.0	Other (or Unknown) Substance Withdrawal
292.0	Sedative, Hypnotic, or Anxiolytic Withdrawal
292.11	Amphetamine-Induced Psychotic Disorder, With Delusions
292.11	Cannabis-Induced Psychotic Disorder, With Delusions
292.11	Cocaine-Induced Psychotic Disorder, With Delusions
292.11	Hallucinogen-Induced Psychotic Disorder, With Delusions
292.11	Inhalant-Induced Psychotic Disorder, With Delusions
292.11	Opioid-Induced Psychotic Disorder, With Delusions
292.11	Other (or Unknown) Substance-Induced Psychotic Disorder, With Delusions
292.11	Phencyclidine-Induced Psychotic Disorder, With Delusions

292.11   Sedative-, Hypnotic-, or Anxiolytic-Induced Psychotic Disorder, With Delusions
292.12   Amphetamine-Induced Psychotic Disorder, With Hallucinations
292.12   Cannabis-Induced Psychotic Disorder, With Hallucinations
292.12   Cocaine-Induced Psychotic Disorder, With Hallucinations
292.12   Hallucinogen-Induced Psychotic Disorder, With Hallucinations
292.12   Inhalant-Induced Psychotic Disorder, With Hallucinations
292.12   Opioid-Induced Psychotic Disorder, With Hallucinations
292.12   Other (or Unknown) Substance-Induced Psychotic Disorder, With Hallucinations
292.12   Phencyclidine-Induced Psychotic Disorder, With Hallucinations
292.12   Sedative-, Hypnotic-, or Anxiolytic-Induced Psychotic Disorder, With Hallucinations
292.81   Amphetamine Intoxication Delirium
292.81   Cannabis Intoxication Delirium
292.81   Cocaine Intoxication Delirium
292.81   Hallucinogen Intoxication Delirium
292.81   Inhalant Intoxication Delirium
292.81   Opioid Intoxication Delirium
292.81   Other (or Unknown) Substance-Induced Delirium
292.81   Phencyclidine Intoxication Delirium
292.81   Sedative, Hypnotic, or Anxiolytic Intoxication Delirium
292.81   Sedative, Hypnotic, or Anxiolytic Withdrawal Delirium
292.82   Inhalant-Induced Persisting Dementia
292.82   Other (or Unknown) Substance-Induced Persisting Dementia
292.82   Sedative-, Hypnotic-, or Anxiolytic-Induced Persisting Dementia
292.83   Other (or Unknown) Substance-Induced Persisting Amnestic Disorder
292.83   Sedative-, Hypnotic-, or Anxiolytic-Induced Persisting Amnestic Disorder
292.84   Amphetamine-Induced Mood Disorder
292.84   Cocaine-Induced Mood Disorder
292.84   Hallucinogen-Induced Mood Disorder
292.84   Inhalant-Induced Mood Disorder
292.84   Opioid-Induced Mood Disorder
292.84   Other (or Unknown) Substance-Induced Mood Disorder
292.84   Phencyclidine-Induced Mood Disorder
292.84   Sedative-, Hypnotic-, or Anxiolytic-Induced Mood Disorder
292.89   Amphetamine-Induced Anxiety Disorder
292.89   Amphetamine-Induced Sexual Dysfunction
292.89   Amphetamine-Induced Sleep Disorder
292.89   Amphetamine Intoxication
292.89   Caffeine-Induced Anxiety Disorder
292.89   Caffeine-Induced Sleep Disorder
292.89   Cannabis-Induced Anxiety Disorder
292.89   Cannabis Intoxication
292.89   Cocaine-Induced Anxiety Disorder

292.89   Cocaine-Induced Sexual Dysfunction
292.89   Cocaine-Induced Sleep Disorder
292.89   Cocaine Intoxication
292.89   Hallucinogen-Induced Anxiety Disorder
292.89   Hallucinogen Intoxication
292.89   Hallucinogen Persisting Perception Disorder
292.89   Inhalant-Induced Anxiety Disorder
292.89   Inhalant Intoxication
292.89   Opioid-Induced Sexual Dysfunction
292.89   Opioid-Induced Sleep Disorder
292.89   Opioid Intoxication
292.89   Other (or Unknown) Substance-Induced Anxiety Disorder
292.89   Other (or Unknown) Substance-Induced Sexual Dysfunction
292.89   Other (or Unknown) Substance-Induced Sleep Disorder
292.89   Other (or Unknown) Substance Intoxication
292.89   Phencyclidine-Induced Anxiety Disorder
292.89   Phencyclidine Intoxication
292.89   Sedative-, Hypnotic-, or Anxiolytic-Induced Anxiety Disorder
292.89   Sedative-, Hypnotic-, or Anxiolytic-Induced Sexual Dysfunction
292.89   Sedative-, Hypnotic-, or Anxiolytic-Induced Sleep Disorder
292.89   Sedative, Hypnotic, or Anxiolytic Intoxication
292.9   Amphetamine-Related Disorder NOS
292.9   Caffeine-Related Disorder NOS
292.9   Cannabis-Related Disorder NOS
292.9   Cocaine-Related Disorder NOS
292.9   Hallucinogen-Related Disorder NOS
292.9   Inhalant-Related Disorder NOS
292.9   Nicotine-Related Disorder NOS
292.9   Opioid-Related Disorder NOS
292.9   Other (or Unknown) Substance-Related Disorder NOS
292.9   Phencyclidine-Related Disorder NOS
292.9   Sedative-, Hypnotic-, or Anxiolytic-Related Disorder NOS
293.0   Delirium Due to . . . [Indicate the General Medical Condition]
293.81   Psychotic Disorder Due to . . . [Indicate the General Medical Condition], With Delusions
293.82   Psychotic Disorder Due to . . . [Indicate the General Medical Condition], With Hallucinations
293.83   Mood Disorder Due to . . . [Indicate the General Medical Condition]
293.84   Anxiety Disorder Due to . . . [Indicate the General Medical Condition]
293.89   Catatonic Disorder Due to . . . [Indicate the General Medical Condition]
293.9   Mental Disorder NOS Due to . . . [Indicate the General Medical Condition]
294.0   Amnestic Disorder Due to . . . [Indicate the General Medical Condition]
294.10   Dementia Due to . . . [Indicate the General Medical Condition], Without Behavioral Disturbance

294.10	Dementia of the Alzheimer's Type, With Early Onset, Without Behavioral Disturbance
294.10	Dementia of the Alzheimer's Type, With Late Onset, Without Behavioral Disturbance
294.11	Dementia Due to . . . [Indicate the General Medical Condition], With Behavioral Disturbance
294.11	Dementia of the Alzheimer's Type, With Early Onset, With Behavioral Disturbance
294.11	Dementia of the Alzheimer's Type, With Late Onset, With Behavioral Disturbance
294.8	Amnestic Disorder NOS
294.8	Dementia NOS
294.9	Cognitive Disorder NOS
295.10	Schizophrenia, Disorganized Type
295.20	Schizophrenia, Catatonic Type
295.30	Schizophrenia, Paranoid Type
295.40	Schizophreniform Disorder
295.60	Schizophrenia, Residual Type
295.70	Schizoaffective Disorder
295.90	Schizophrenia, Undifferentiated Type
296.00	Bipolar I Disorder, Single Manic Episode, Unspecified
296.01	Bipolar I Disorder, Single Manic Episode, Mild
296.02	Bipolar I Disorder, Single Manic Episode, Moderate
296.03	Bipolar I Disorder, Single Manic Episode, Severe Without Psychotic Features
296.04	Bipolar I Disorder, Single Manic Episode, Severe With Psychotic Features
296.05	Bipolar I Disorder, Single Manic Episode, In Partial Remission
296.06	Bipolar I Disorder, Single Manic Episode, In Full Remission
296.20	Major Depressive Disorder, Single Episode, Unspecified
296.21	Major Depressive Disorder, Single Episode, Mild
296.22	Major Depressive Disorder, Single Episode, Moderate
296.23	Major Depressive Disorder, Single Episode, Severe Without Psychotic Features
296.24	Major Depressive Disorder, Single Episode, Severe With Psychotic Features
296.25	Major Depressive Disorder, Single Episode, In Partial Remission
296.26	Major Depressive Disorder, Single Episode, In Full Remission
296.30	Major Depressive Disorder, Recurrent, Unspecified
296.31	Major Depressive Disorder, Recurrent, Mild
296.32	Major Depressive Disorder, Recurrent, Moderate
296.33	Major Depressive Disorder, Recurrent, Severe Without Psychotic Features
296.34	Major Depressive Disorder, Recurrent, Severe With Psychotic Features
296.35	Major Depressive Disorder, Recurrent, In Partial Remission
296.36	Major Depressive Disorder, Recurrent, In Full Remission
296.40	Bipolar I Disorder, Most Recent Episode Hypomanic
296.40	Bipolar I Disorder, Most Recent Episode Manic, Unspecified
296.41	Bipolar I Disorder, Most Recent Episode Manic, Mild

296.42	Bipolar I Disorder, Most Recent Episode Manic, Moderate
296.43	Bipolar I Disorder, Most Recent Episode Manic, Severe Without Psychotic Features
296.44	Bipolar I Disorder, Most Recent Episode Manic, Severe With Psychotic Features
296.45	Bipolar I Disorder, Most Recent Episode Manic, In Partial Remission
296.46	Bipolar I Disorder, Most Recent Episode Manic, In Full Remission
296.50	Bipolar I Disorder, Most Recent Episode Depressed, Unspecified
296.51	Bipolar I Disorder, Most Recent Episode Depressed, Mild
296.52	Bipolar I Disorder, Most Recent Episode Depressed, Moderate
296.53	Bipolar I Disorder, Most Recent Episode Depressed, Severe Without Psychotic Features
296.54	Bipolar I Disorder, Most Recent Episode Depressed, Severe With Psychotic Features
296.55	Bipolar I Disorder, Most Recent Episode Depressed, In Partial Remission
296.56	Bipolar I Disorder, Most Recent Episode Depressed, In Full Remission
296.60	Bipolar I Disorder, Most Recent Episode Mixed, Unspecified
296.61	Bipolar I Disorder, Most Recent Episode Mixed, Mild
296.62	Bipolar I Disorder, Most Recent Episode Mixed, Moderate
296.63	Bipolar I Disorder, Most Recent Episode Mixed, Severe Without Psychotic Features
296.64	Bipolar I Disorder, Most Recent Episode Mixed, Severe With Psychotic Features
296.65	Bipolar I Disorder, Most Recent Episode Mixed, In Partial Remission
296.66	Bipolar I Disorder, Most Recent Episode Mixed, In Full Remission
296.7	Bipolar I Disorder, Most Recent Episode Unspecified
296.80	Bipolar Disorder NOS
296.89	Bipolar II Disorder
296.90	Mood Disorder NOS
297.1	Delusional Disorder
297.3	Shared Psychotic Disorder
298.8	Brief Psychotic Disorder
298.9	Psychotic Disorder NOS
299.00	Autistic Disorder
299.10	Childhood Disintegrative Disorder
299.80	Asperger's Disorder
299.80	Pervasive Developmental Disorder NOS
299.80	Rett's Disorder
300.00	Anxiety Disorder NOS
300.01	Panic Disorder Without Agoraphobia
300.02	Generalized Anxiety Disorder
300.11	Conversion Disorder
300.12	Dissociative Amnesia
300.13	Dissociative Fugue
300.14	Dissociative Identity Disorder

300.15	Dissociative Disorder NOS
300.16	Factitious Disorder With Predominantly Psychological Signs and Symptoms
300.19	Factitious Disorder NOS
300.19	Factitious Disorder With Combined Psychological and Physical Signs and Symptoms
300.19	Factitious Disorder With Predominantly Physical Signs and Symptoms
300.21	Panic Disorder With Agoraphobia
300.22	Agoraphobia Without History of Panic Disorder
300.23	Social Phobia
300.29	Specific Phobia
300.3	Obsessive-Compulsive Disorder
300.4	Dysthymic Disorder
300.6	Depersonalization Disorder
300.7	Body Dysmorphic Disorder
300.7	Hypochondriasis
300.81	Somatization Disorder
300.82	Somatoform Disorder NOS
300.82	Undifferentiated Somatoform Disorder
300.9	Unspecified Mental Disorder (nonpsychotic)
301.0	Paranoid Personality Disorder
301.13	Cyclothymic Disorder
301.20	Schizoid Personality Disorder
301.22	Schizotypal Personality Disorder
301.4	Obsessive-Compulsive Personality Disorder
301.50	Histrionic Personality Disorder
301.6	Dependent Personality Disorder
301.7	Antisocial Personality Disorder
301.81	Narcissistic Personality Disorder
301.82	Avoidant Personality Disorder
301.83	Borderline Personality Disorder
301.9	Personality Disorder NOS
302.2	Pedophilia
302.3	Transvestic Fetishism
302.4	Exhibitionism
302.6	Gender Identity Disorder in Children
302.6	Gender Identity Disorder NOS
302.70	Sexual Dysfunction NOS
302.71	Hypoactive Sexual Desire Disorder
302.72	Female Sexual Arousal Disorder
302.72	Male Erectile Disorder
302.73	Female Orgasmic Disorder
302.74	Male Orgasmic Disorder
302.75	Premature Ejaculation
302.76	Dyspareunia (Not Due to a General Medical Condition)
302.79	Sexual Aversion Disorder

302.81	Fetishism
302.82	Voyeurism
302.83	Sexual Masochism
302.84	Sexual Sadism
302.85	Gender Identity Disorder in Adolescents or Adults
302.89	Frotteurism
302.9	Paraphilia NOS
302.9	Sexual Disorder NOS
303.00	Alcohol Intoxication
303.90	Alcohol Dependence
304.00	Opioid Dependence
304.10	Sedative, Hypnotic, or Anxiolytic Dependence
304.20	Cocaine Dependence
304.30	Cannabis Dependence
304.40	Amphetamine Dependence
304.50	Hallucinogen Dependence
304.60	Inhalant Dependence
304.60	Phencyclidine Dependence
304.80	Polysubstance Dependence
304.90	Other (or Unknown) Substance Dependence
305.00	Alcohol Abuse
305.1	Nicotine Dependence
305.20	Cannabis Abuse
305.30	Hallucinogen Abuse
305.40	Sedative, Hypnotic, or Anxiolytic Abuse
305.50	Opioid Abuse
305.60	Cocaine Abuse
305.70	Amphetamine Abuse
305.90	Caffeine Intoxication
305.90	Inhalant Abuse
305.90	Other (or Unknown) Substance Abuse
305.90	Phencyclidine Abuse
306.51	Vaginismus (Not Due to a General Medical Condition)
307.0	Stuttering
307.1	Anorexia Nervosa
307.20	Tic Disorder NOS
307.21	Transient Tic Disorder
307.22	Chronic Motor or Vocal Tic Disorder
307.23	Tourette's Disorder
307.3	Stereotypic Movement Disorder
307.42	Insomnia Related to . . . [Indicate the Axis I or Axis II Disorder]
307.42	Primary Insomnia
307.44	Hypersomnia Related to . . . [Indicate the Axis I or Axis II Disorder]
307.44	Primary Hypersomnia
307.45	Circadian Rhythm Sleep Disorder

307.46	Sleep Terror Disorder
307.46	Sleepwalking Disorder
307.47	Dyssomnia NOS
307.47	Nightmare Disorder
307.47	Parasomnia NOS
307.50	Eating Disorder NOS
307.51	Bulimia Nervosa
307.52	Pica
307.53	Rumination Disorder
307.59	Feeding Disorder of Infancy or Early Childhood
307.6	Enuresis (Not Due to a General Medical Condition)
307.7	Encopresis, Without Constipation and Overflow Incontinence
307.80	Pain Disorder Associated With Psychological Factors
307.89	Pain Disorder Associated With Both Psychological Factors and a General Medical Condition
307.9	Communication Disorder NOS
308.3	Acute Stress Disorder
309.0	Adjustment Disorder With Depressed Mood
309.21	Separation Anxiety Disorder
309.24	Adjustment Disorder With Anxiety
309.28	Adjustment Disorder With Mixed Anxiety and Depressed Mood
309.3	Adjustment Disorder With Disturbance of Conduct
309.4	Adjustment Disorder With Mixed Disturbance of Emotions and Conduct
309.81	Posttraumatic Stress Disorder
309.9	Adjustment Disorder Unspecified
310.1	Personality Change Due to . . . [Indicate the General Medical Condition]
311	Depressive Disorder NOS
312.30	Impulse-Control Disorder NOS
312.31	Pathological Gambling
312.32	Kleptomania
312.33	Pyromania
312.34	Intermittent Explosive Disorder
312.39	Trichotillomania
312.81	Conduct Disorder, Childhood-Onset Type
312.82	Conduct Disorder, Adolescent-Onset Type
312.89	Conduct Disorder, Unspecified Onset
312.9	Disruptive Behavior Disorder NOS
313.23	Selective Mutism
313.81	Oppositional Defiant Disorder
313.82	Identity Problem
313.89	Reactive Attachment Disorder of Infancy or Early Childhood
313.9	Disorder of Infancy, Childhood, or Adolescence NOS
314.00	Attention-Deficit/Hyperactivity Disorder, Predominantly Inattentive Type
314.01	Attention-Deficit/Hyperactivity Disorder, Combined Type

314.01	Attention-Deficit/Hyperactivity Disorder, Predominantly Hyperactive-Impulsive Type
314.9	Attention-Deficit/Hyperactivity Disorder NOS
315.00	Reading Disorder
315.1	Mathematics Disorder
315.2	Disorder of Written Expression
315.31	Expressive Language Disorder
315.32	Mixed Receptive-Expressive Language Disorder
315.39	Phonological Disorder
315.4	Developmental Coordination Disorder
315.9	Learning Disorder NOS
316	. . . [Specified Psychological Factor] Affecting . . . [Indicate the General Medical Condition]
317	Mild Mental Retardation
318.0	Moderate Mental Retardation
318.1	Severe Mental Retardation
318.2	Profound Mental Retardation
319	Mental Retardation, Severity Unspecified
332.1	Neuroleptic-Induced Parkinsonism
333.1	Medication-Induced Postural Tremor
333.7	Neuroleptic-Induced Acute Dystonia
333.82	Neuroleptic-Induced Tardive Dyskinesia
333.90	Medication-Induced Movement Disorder NOS
333.92	Neuroleptic Malignant Syndrome
333.99	Neuroleptic-Induced Acute Akathisia
347	Narcolepsy
607.84	Male Erectile Disorder Due to . . . [Indicate the General Medical Condition]
608.89	Male Dyspareunia Due to . . . [Indicate the General Medical Condition]
608.89	Male Hypoactive Sexual Desire Disorder Due to . . . [Indicate the Medical Condition]
608.89	Other Male Sexual Dysfunction Due to . . . [Indicate the General Medical Condition]
625.0	Female Dyspareunia Due to . . . [Indicate the General Medical Condition]
625.8	Female Hypoactive Sexual Desire Disorder Due to . . . [Indicate the General Medical Condition]
625.8	Other Female Sexual Dysfunction Due to . . . [Indicate the General Medical Condition]
780.09	Delirium NOS
780.52	Sleep Disorder Due to . . . [Indicate the General Medical Condition], Insomnia Type
780.54	Sleep Disorder Due to . . . [Indicate the General Medical Condition], Hypersomnia Type
780.59	Breathing-Related Sleep Disorder
780.59	Sleep Disorder Due to . . . [Indicate the General Medical Condition], Mixed Type

780.59	Sleep Disorder Due to . . . [Indicate the General Medical Condition], Parasomnia Type
780.9	Age-Related Cognitive Decline
787.6	Encopresis, With Constipation and Overflow Incontinence
799.9	Diagnosis Deferred on Axis II
799.9	Diagnosis or Condition Deferred on Axis I
995.2	Adverse Effects of Medication NOS
995.52	Neglect of Child (if focus of attention is on victim)
995.53	Sexual Abuse of Child (if focus of attention is on victim)
995.54	Physical Abuse of Child (if focus of attention is on victim)
995.81	Physical Abuse of Adult (if focus of attention is on victim)
995.83	Sexual Abuse of Adult (if focus of attention is on victim)
V15.81	Noncompliance With Treatment
V61.10	Partner Relational Problem
V61.12	Physical Abuse of Adult (if by partner)
V61.12	Sexual Abuse of Adult (if by partner)
V61.20	Parent-Child Relational Problem
V61.21	Neglect of Child
V61.21	Physical Abuse of Child
V61.21	Sexual Abuse of Child
V61.8	Sibling Relational Problem
V61.9	Relational Problem Related to a Mental Disorder or General Medical Condition
V62.2	Occupational Problem
V62.3	Academic Problem
V62.4	Acculturation Problem
V62.81	Relational Problem NOS
V62.82	Bereavement
V62.83	Physical Abuse of Adult (if by person other than partner)
V62.83	Sexual Abuse of Adult (if by person other than partner)
V62.89	Borderline Intellectual Functioning
V62.89	Phase of Life Problem
V62.89	Religious or Spiritual Problem
V65.2	Malingering
V71.01	Adult Antisocial Behavior
V71.02	Child or Adolescent Antisocial Behavior
V71.09	No Diagnosis on Axis II
V71.09	No Diagnosis or Condition on Axis I

Appendix B
Listing of Advocacy and
Self-Help Resources

Chapter 1
Disorders Usually First Diagnosed in Infancy,
Childhood, or Adolescence

Section 1: Mental Retardation

Advocacy/Support Organizations

Association for Retarded Citizens
1010 Wayne Ave., Suite 650   301-565-3842
Silver Spring, MD 20910   http://www.thearc.org/

National Down-Syndrome Congress
1605 Chantilly Drive, Suite 250   404-633-2817
Atlanta, GA 30324   800-232-NDSC

National Down-Syndrome Society   212-460-9330
666 Broadway   800-221-4602
New York, NY 10012   http://www.ndss.org

The National Fragile X Foundation   510-763-6030
P.O. Box 190488   800-688-8765
San Francisco, CA 94119   http://www.fragilex.org

Videos

Organizations listed under Advocacy/Support may also have videos—see their Web sites.

Books

McNey, Martha, and Leslie Fish. *Leslie's Story: A Book about a Girl with Mental Retardation*.
    Minneapolis, MN: Lerner Publications, 1996.

Section 2: Learning Disorders

Advocacy/Support Organizations

The ERIC Clearinghouse on Disabilities and Gifted Education (ERIC EC)
The Council for Exceptional Children
1920 Association Drive   800-328-0272
Reston, VA 20191   http://www.ericec.org

Learning Disabilities Association of America
4156 Library Road
Pittsburgh, PA 15234   412-341-1515

Section 5: Pervasive Developmental Disorders

Advocacy/Support Organizations
Autism Society of America   301-657-0881
7910 Woodmont Avenue, Suite 650   800-3-AUTISM
Bethesda, MD 20814   http://www.autism-society.org

Online Asperger Syndrome Information & Support Group™
(O.A.S.I.S.)   http://www.udel.edu.bkirby/asperger

Videos/Movies
Rain Man (Dustin Hoffman as Raymond Babbitt). MGM/Universal Artist Studios, 1988.
    Filmstrip.

Books
Williams, Donna. *Nobody Nowhere: The Extraordinary Autobiography of an Autistic*. New York,
    NY: Avon Books, 1994.

Section 6: Attention-Deficit and Disruptive Behavior Disorders

Advocacy/Support Organizations
Children and Adults with Attention-Deficit/Hyperactivity
    Disorder (CHADD)   800-233-4060
499 North Seventieth Avenue, Suite 109   954-587-3700
Plantation, FL 33317   http://www.chadd.org/

National ADDA
1070 Rosewood Avenue, Suite A   800-497-2282, 800-975-0004, 440-350-9595
Ann Arbor, MI 48104   http://www.add.org/

Toughlove
P.O. Box 1069   800-333-1069
Doylestown, PA 18901   http://www.toughlove.org/

Books
Wender, Paul H. *Attention-Deficit Hyperactivity Disorder in Adults*. New York, NY: Oxford
    University Press, 1995.

Section 8: Tic Disorders

Advocacy/Support Organizations
Tourette Syndrome Association, Inc.
42-40 Bell Boulevard, Suite 205   888-4-TOURET
Bayside, NY 11361   http://www.tsa-usa.org

Videos
The Tic Code (Christopher Marquette as Miles; Gregory Hines as Tyrone). Avalanche Releasing, 2000.

Books
Leckman, James F., and Donald J. Cohen. *Tourette's Syndrome: Tics, Obsessions, Compulsions*, 1st edition. New York, NY: John Wiley and Sons, Inc., 1998.

Section 9: Elimination Disorders

Advocacy/Support Organizations
National Eneuresis Society
7777 Forest Lane, Suite C-737
Dallas, TX 75230-2518

800-NES-8080
http://www.peds.umn.edu/Centers/NES/

Chapter 2
Delirium, Dementia, Amnestic, and Other Cognitive Disorders

Section 2: Dementia

Advocacy/Support Organizations
Alzheimer's Disease and Related Disorders Association
919 North Michigan Avenue, Suite 1000
Chicago, IL 60611-1676

312-335-8700
800-572-6037
http://www.alzheimers.org/

National Family Caregivers Association
10605 Concord Street, Suite 501
Kensington, MD 20895-2504

800-896-3650
http://www.nfcacares.org

National Stroke Association
96 Inverness Drive, East, Suite One
Englewood, CO 80112-5112

303-649-9299
http://www.stroke.org

Videos
APA videos—see p. 125.

Books
Hay, Jennifer. *Alzheimer's and Dementia: Questions You Have . . . Answers You Need.* Allentown, PA: People's Medical Society, 1996.
Mace, Nancy L., and Peter V. Rabins. *The 36-Hour Day: A Family Guide on Caring for Persons with Alzheimer's Disease, Related Dementing Illness and Memory Loss in Later Life*, 3rd edition, Baltimore, MD: Johns Hopkins University, 1999.

Section 4: Postconcussional Disorder

Advocacy/Support Organizations
The Brain Injury Association, Inc.
105 North Alfred Street   703-236-6000
Alexandria, VA 22314   http://www.biausa.org/

Chapter 3
Substance-Related Disorders

Section 1: Dependence and Abuse

Advocacy/Support Organizations
Al-Anon, Alateen, Adult Children of Alcoholics
Al-Anon Family Group Headquarters, Inc.
1600 Corporate Landing Parkway   757-563-1600
Virginia Beach, VA 23454-5617   http://www.al-anon.alateen.org/

Alcoholics Anonymous World Services, Inc.
P.O. Box 459
Grand Central Station   212-870-3400
New York, NY 10163   http://www.alcoholics-anonymous.org/

Cocaine Anonymous World Services
P.O. Box 2000   310-559-5833
Los Angeles, CA 90049-8000   http://www.ca.org/

Families Anonymous—World Service Office
Box 3475
Culver City, CA 90231-3475   800-736-9805

Marijuana Anonymous
P.O. Box 2912   800-766-6779
Van Nuys, CA 91404   http://www.marijuana-anonymous.org/

Narcotics Anonymous
P.O. Box 9999   818-773-9999
Van Nuys, CA 91409   http://www.na.org/

National Council on Alcoholism and Drug Dependence, Inc.
12 West 21st Street   212-206-6770
New York, NY 10010   http://www.ncadd.org

Women for Sobriety, Inc.
P.O. Box 618   800-333-1606
Quakerstown, PA 18951   215-536-8026

Videos/Movies
APA videos—see p. 125.

Organizations listed under *Advocacy/Support* may also have videos—see their Web sites.

Books

Cheever, Susan. *Note Found in a Bottle: My Life as a Drinker*. New York, NY: Simon & Schuster, 1999.

McCourt, Frank. *Angela's Ashes: A Memoir*. New York, NY: Scribner, 1996.

Chapter 4
Schizophrenia and Other Psychotic Disorders

Advocacy/Support Organizations

National Alliance for the Mentally Ill
200 N. Glebe Rd., Suite 1015   800-950-NAMI
Arlington, VA 22203-3754   http://www.nami.org

National Alliance for Research on Schizophrenia and Depression (NARSAD)
60 Cutter Mill Road, Suite 404   516-829-0091
Great Neck, NY 11021   http://www.mhsource.com/narsad

National Mental Health Association   703-684-7722
1021 Prince Street   800-969-NMHA
Alexandria, VA 22314-2971   http://www.nmha.org

National Mental Health Consumers' Self-Help Clearing House
1211 Chestnut Street, Suite 1207   800-553-4539
Philadelphia, PA 19107   http://www.mhselfhelp.org

On Our Own
213 Monroe Street
Rockville, MD 20850   301-251-3734

Recovery Inc.
802 Dearborn St.   312-337-5661
Chicago, IL 60610   http://www.recovery-inc.com

Schizophrenics Anonymous
15920 W. Twelve Mile   800-482-9534
Southfield, MI 48076   http://www.sanonymous.org

Videos/Movies
APA videos—see p. 125.

Organizations listed under *Advocacy/Support* may also have videos—see their Web sites.

Books

Burke, Ross, and David Burke. *When the Music's Over: My Journey into Schizophrenia*. Editors, Richard Gates and Robin Hammond, New York, NY: Plume, 1996.

Greenberg, Joanne. *I Never Promised You a Rose Garden*. New York, NY: Holt, Rinehart and Winston, 1964.

Holley, Tara Elgin, and Joe Holley. *My Mother's Keeper: A Daughter's Memoir of Growing Up in the Shadow of Schizophrenia*, 1st edition. New York, NY: W. Morrow, 1997.

Chapter 5
Mood Disorders

Section 1: Depressive Disorders

Advocacy/Support Organizations

American Foundation for Suicide Prevention
120 Wall Street, 22nd Floor   888-333-AFSP
New York, NY 10005   http://www.afsp.org

Depression After Delivery
P.O. Box 1282   1-800-944-4773
Morrisville, PA 19607   http://www.behavenet.com/dadinc/

Depression & Related Affective Disorders Association (DRADA)
Johns Hopkins Hospital
Meyer 3-181
600 North Wolfe Street   410-955-4647
Baltimore, MD 21287-7381   http://www.med.jhu.edu/drada

National Alliance for the Mentally Ill (NAMI)
200 North Glebe Road, Suite 1015   1-800-950-6264
Arlington, VA 22203-3754   http://www.nami.org

National Depressive and Manic Depressive Association
730 N. Franklin, Suite 501   800-826-3632
Chicago, IL 60610-3526   http://www.ndmda.org

National Mental Health Association
1021 Prince Street   1-800-969-NMHA
Alexandria, VA 22314-2971   http://www.nmha.org

Videos/Movies

Day for Night: Recognizing Teenage Depression (26 minute video), produced by DRADA, 1999. 410-955-4647.

Books

Danquah, Meri Nana-Ama. *Willow Weep for Me: A Black Woman's Journey through Depression: A Memoir*. New York, NY: Norton, 1999.

Jamison, Kay Redfield. *Night Falls Fast: Understanding Suicide*. New York, NY: Knopf, 1999.

Styron, William. *Darkness Visible: A Memoir of Madness*. New York, NY: Vintage Books, 1992.

Section 2: Bipolar Disorders

Advocacy/Support Organizations

See listings under Section 1.

Books

Jamison, Kay Redfield. *An Unquiet Mind*. New York, NY: Vintage Books, 1996.

————. *Touched with Fire: Manic-Depressive Illness and the Artistic Temperament*. New York, NY: The Free Press, 1996.

Chapter 6
Anxiety Disorders

Advocacy/Support Organizations

Anxiety Disorders Association of America
11900 Parklawn Drive, Suite 100
Rockville, MD 20852-2624   http://www.adaa.org

Dale Carnegie Training
1475 Franklin Avenue   800-231-5800
Garden City, NY 11530   http://www.DaleCarnegie.com

Freedom From Fear
308 Seaview Ave.
Staten Island, NY 10305   http://www.freedomfromfear.org

National Alliance for the Mentally Ill (NAMI)
200 North Glebe Road, Suite 1015   1-800-950-6264
Arlington, VA 22203-3754   http://www.nami.org

National Mental Health Association (NMHA)
1021 Prince Street
Alexandria, VA 22314-2971   800-969-NMHA

National Speaker Association
1500 South Priest Drive
Tempe, AZ 85281   http://www.speaker.org

Toastmasters
Toastmasters International
23182 Arroyo Vista   949-858-8255
Rancho Santa Margarita, CA 92688   http://www.toastmasters.org

Videos/Movies
APA videos—see p. 125.

Books
Ross, Jerilyn. *Triumph over Fear: A Book of Help and Hope for People with Anxiety, Panic Attacks, and Phobias*, with foreword by Rosalynn Carter. New York, NY: Bantam Books, 1994.

Section 1: Panic Disorder and Phobias

Advocacy/Support Organizations
Agoraphobics in Motion (A.I.M.)
1719 Crooks
Royal Oak, MI 48067   248-547-0400

Phobics Anonymous
P.O. Box 1180
Palm Springs, CA 92263   619-322-COPE (2673)

Books
Poe, Edgar Allan. "The Telltale Heart and The Cask of Amontillado," published in *Godey's Lady's Book*. 1846.

Section 2: Obsessive-Compulsive Disorder

Advocacy/Support Organizations
The Obsessive Compulsive Foundation, Inc.
P.O. 9573   203-315-2190
New Haven, CT 06535   http://www.ocfoundation.org

Videos/Movies
As Good As It Gets (Jack Nicholson as Melvin Udall). Columbia/Tristar Studios, 1997. Filmstrip.

APA videos—see p. 125.

Books
Shakespeare, William. *Macbeth* (Lady Macbeth).

Section 3: Posttraumatic Stress Disorder

Advocacy/Support Organizations (*also see* Chapter 14, "Adjustment Disorders" *resources*)
American Medical Association Violence Prevention Web Site
                                            http://www.ama-assn.org/violence

International Society for Traumatic Stress Studies (ISTSS)
60 Revere Drive, Suite 500
Northbrook, IL 60062

National Center for Posttraumatic Stress Disorder (PTSD)
215 N. Main Street 802-296-5132
White River Junction, VT 05009 http://www.dartmouth.edu/dms/ptsd

The Sidran Foundation and Press
200 East Joppa Road, Suite 207 410-825-8888
Baltimore, MD 21286 E-mail: sidran@sidran.org

Veterans Administration
Veterans Health Administration
1120 Vermont Avenue, NW
Washington, DC 20421 http://www.va.gov/About_VA/Orgs/VHA/VHAProg.htm

Videos/Movies
Ordinary People (Donald Sutherland, Mary Tyler Moore, Timothy Hutton, and Judd Hirsch). Paramount Studio, 1980. Filmstrip.
The Deer Hunter (Robert De Niro, John Savage, and Christopher Walken). Universal Studios, 1978. Filmstrip.

APA videos—see p. 125.

Books
Levi, Primo. *Survival in Auschwitz: The Nazi Assault on Humanity*. New York, NY: Collier Books, 1995.
Styron, William. *Sophie's Choice*. New York, NY: Modern Library, 1999.

Section 4: Generalized Anxiety Disorder

Videos/Movies
Annie Hall (Woody Allen and Diane Keaton). MGM/UA Studios, 1977. Filmstrip.
A Streetcar Named Desire (character of Blanche DuBois). Tennessee Williams. Warner Studios, 1951, 1984, 1995. Filmstrip.

Chapter 7
Somatoform Disorders

Section 2: Conversion Disorder

Books
Freud, Sigmund. "Frau Emmy Von N" *The Standard Edition of the Complete Psychological Works of Sigmund Freud*, Vol. II, translated by James Strachey. London, England: Hogarth Press, 1955.
Williams, Tennesee. *Cat on a Hot Tin Roof*. New York, NY: New Directions, 1955.

Section 3: Pain Disorder

Advocacy/Support Organizations
American Chronic Pain Association
P.O. Box 850   916-632-0922
Rocklin, CA 95677   http://www.members.tripod.com/-Widdy/ACPA.html

Books
Aeschylus. *Prometheus Bound*, play, 5th Century B.C.
Shelley, Percy Bysshe. *Prometheus Unbound*, lyrical drama, 1820.

Section 4: Hypochondriasis

Books
Aesop. *Shepherd Boy and the Wolf*, fable, 6th Century B.C.
Cantor, Carla, and Brian Fallon. *Phantom Illness: Recognizing, Understanding, and Overcoming Hypochondria, Shattering the Myths of Hypochondria*. Boston, MA: Houghton Mifflin, 1997.

Section 5: Body Dysmorphic Disorder

Books
Rostand, Edmond. *Cyrano de Bergerac*, play, 1897.
Andersen, Hans Christian. *The Ugly Duckling*, fairy tale, 19th Century.

Chapter 9
Dissociative Disorders

Section 3: Dissociative Identity Disorder

Advocacy/Support Organizations
The Sidran Foundation and Press
200 East Joppa Road, Suite 207   410-825-8888
Baltimore, MD 21286   E-mail: sidran@sidran.org

Videos
Phoenix J. Hocking. *37 to One: Living as an Integrated Multiple*. Brandon, VT: The Safer Society Press, 1996. Video.

Books
Cohen, Barry M., Esther Giller, and Lynn W., eds. *Multiple Personality Disorder from the Inside Out*. Baltimore, MD: Sidran Press, 1991.
Sessions, Deborah. *My Mom Is Different*, illustrated by Susan Chalkley. Baltimore, MD: Sidran Press, 1994.

Chapter 10
Sexual and Gender Identity Disorders

Section 1: Sexual Dysfunction

Advocacy/Support Organizations
Impotence Information Center
P.O. Box 9   800-843-4315
Minneapolis, MN 55440

Sexual Information & Education Council of the United States
The Mary S. Calderone Library
130 West 42nd Street, Suite 350   212-819-9717
New York, NY 10036-7802   http://www.siecus.org

Section 2: Paraphilia

Advocacy/Support Organizations
The Safer Society Foundation, Inc.
P.O. Box 340
Brandon, VT 05733-0340   802-247-3132

Videos/Movies
APA videos—see p. 125.

Boys Don't Cry (character of Brandon Teena). CBS/Fox Home Video, 1999.

Books
Heiman, Julia, and Joseph Lopiccolo. *Becoming Orgasmic: A Sexual and Personal Growth Program for Women*. New York, NY: Prentice Hall, 1988.
Reinisch, June M., and Ruth Beasley. *The Kinsey Institute New Report on Sex: What You Must Know to Be Sexually Literate*. New York, NY: St. Martin's Press, Inc., 1991.

Chapter 11
Eating Disorders

Section 1: Anorexia Nervosa

Advocacy/Support Organizations
American Anorexia/Bulimia Association, Inc.
165 West 46th Street, Suite 1108   212-575-6200
New York, NY 10036   http://www.aabainc.org

Eating Disorders Awareness & Prevention
National Association of Anorexia Nervosa and Associated Disorders
Box 7   847-831-3438
Highland Park, IL 60035   http://www.anad.org

National Eating Disorder Organization
603 Stewart Street, Suite 803
Seattle, WA 98101   http://www.EDAP.org

Books
Bruch, Hilde. *The Golden Cage: The Enigma of Anorexia Nervosa.* New York, NY: Vintage Books,
    1979.
Brumberg, Joan Jacobs. *The Body Project: An Intimate History of American Girls.* New York, NY:
    Vintage Books, 1998.
Lemberg, Raymond, ed. *Eating Disorders: A Reference Sourcebook*, ed. Phoenix, AZ: Oryx Press,
    1999.

Section 2: Bulimia Nervosa

Advocacy/Support Organizations
S.M.A.R.T. Recovery Self-Help Network
(Self-Management & Recovery Training)
24000 Mercantile Road, Suite 33   440-951-5357
Beachwood, OH 44122   http://www.smartrecovery.org

Videos
APA videos—see p. 125.

Organizations listed under *Advocacy/Support* may also have videos—see their Web sites.

Books
Hornbacher, Marya. *Wasted: A Memoir of Anorexia and Bulimia.* New York, NY: HarperCollins
    Publishers, 1998.

Chapter 12
Sleep Disorders

Advocacy/Support Organizations
Narcolepsy Network
10921 Reed Hartman Highway, Suite 19   Fax: 513-891-3522
Cincinnati, OH 45242   E-mail: Narnet@aol.com

National Sleep Foundation
729 15th Street, NW, Fourth Floor   202-347-3471
Washington, DC 20005   http://www.sleepfoundation.org/

Books

Dement, William C., and Christopher Vaughan. *The Promise of Sleep: A Pioneer in Sleep Medicine Explains the Vital Connection between Health, Happiness and a Good Sleep.* New York, NY: Delacorte Press, 1999.

Hauri, Peter, and Shirley Linde. *No More Sleepless Nights*, revised edition. New York, NY: John Wiley and Sons, Inc., 1996.

Chapter 13
Impulse-Control Disorders

Section 1: Intermittent Explosive Disorder

Advocacy/Support Organizations *(also see* Chapter 14, "Adjustment Disorders" *resources)*

Center for the Prevention of School Violence
313 Chapanoke Road, Suite 140   800-299-6054
Raleigh, NC 27603   http://www.ncsu.edu/cpsv/

Videos/Movies

American History X (Stacy Keach, Fairuzza Balk, Beverly D'Angelo, Elliott Gould, and Avery Brooks), Edward Norton, Edward Furlong. New Line Productions, 1998.

Books

Bodine, Richard J., and Donna K. Crawford. *The Handbook of Conflict Resolution Education: A Guide to Building Quality Programs in Schools.* San Francisco, CA: Jossey-Bass Publishers, 1997.

Flannery, Raymond B. *Preventing Youth Violence: A Guide for Parents, Teachers, and Counselors.* New York, NY: Continuum Publishing Group, 1999.

Garbarino, James. *Lost Boys: Why Our Sons Turn Violent and How We Can Save Them.* New York, NY: The Free Press, 1999.

Section 2: Kleptomania

Advocacy/Support Organizations

Shoplifters Alternative
380 N. Broadway   888-466-2299
Jericho, NY 11753   http://www.shopliftersalternative.org

Videos/Movies

Marnie (Tippy Hedren and Sean Connery). Universal Studios, 1964. Filmstrip (rated PG).

Books

Goldman, Marcus J. *Kleptomania: The Compulsion to Steal—What Can Be Done.* Far Hills, NJ: New Horizon Press, 1999.

Cupchik, Will. *Why Honest People Shoplift or Commit Other Acts of Theft: Assessment and Treatment of 'Atypical Theft Offenders.'* Toronto, ON: University of Toronto Press, 1997.

Section 3: Pyromania

Advocacy/Support Organizations
The United States Fire Administration (USFA)
Office of Fire Management Programs
16825 South Seton Avenue
Emmitsburg, MD 21727   www.usfa.fema.gov

Books
Fitch, Richard D., and Edward A. Porter. *Accidental or Incendiary*, 2nd edition. Springfield, IL: Charles C. Thomas Publishing Ltd., 1997.
Sakheim, George A., and Elizabeth Osborn. *Firesetting Children: Risk Assessment and Treatment.* Washington, DC: Child Welfare League of America, 1994.

Section 4: Pathological Gambling

Advocacy/Support Organizations
Gam-Anon International Service Office, Inc.
(for families and spouses)
P.O. Box 157   718-352-1671
Whitestone, NY 11357   http://www.fam-anon.org/

Gamblers Anonymous
P.O. Box 17173   213-386-8789
Los Angeles, CA 90017   http://www.gamblersanonymous.org/

Videos/Movies
APA videos—see p. 125.

Books
Barthelme, Frederick, and Steven Barthelme. *Double Down: Reflections on Gambling and Loss.* Boston, MA: Houghton Mifflin, 1999.
Haubrich-Casperson, Jane, and Doug Van Nispen. *Coping with Teen Gambling*, 1st edition. New York, NY: The Rosen Publishing Group, 1993.

Section 5: Trichotillomania

Advocacy/Support Organizations
The Obsessive Compulsive Foundation, Inc.
P.O. 9573   203-315-2190
New Haven, CT 06535   http://www.ocfoundation.org

Trichotillomania Learning Center
1215 Mission Street
Santa Cruz, CA 95060

831-457-1004
http://www.trich.org

Books

Golomb, Ruth Goldfinger, and Sherrie Mansfield Vavrichek. *The Hair Pulling Habit and You: How to Solve the Trichotillomania Puzzle*. Washington, DC: Writer's Cooperative of Greater Washington, 1999.

Anders, Jeffrey L., and James W. Jefferson. *Trichotillomania: A Guide*. Madison, WI: Madison Institute of Medicine, 1998.

Chapter 14
Adjustment Disorders

Advocacy/Support Organizations (*also see* Chapter 6, "Posttraumatic Stress Disorders" *resources, and* Chapter 16, "Other Syndromes" *resources*)

American Institute of Stress
124 Park Avenue
Yonkers, NY 10703

914-963-1200
http://www.stress.org

American Medical Association Violence
Prevention Web Site

http://www.ama-assn.org/violence

American Red Cross
Disaster Services
431 18th Street, NW
Washington, DC 20006

202-639-3520
http://www.redcross.org

National Organization for Victim Assistance (NOVA)
1757 Park Road, NW
Washington, DC 20010

800-879-6682
http://www.try-nova.org

Project PAVE (Promoting Alternatives to Violence through Education)
2051 York Street
Denver, CO 80205

303-322-2382

Books

Bodine, Richard J., and Donna K. Crawford. *The Handbook of Conflict Resolution Education: A Guide to Building Quality Programs in Schools*. San Francisco, CA: Jossey-Bass Publishers, 1997.

Flannery, Raymond B. *Preventing Youth Violence: A Guide for Parents, Teachers, and Counselors*. New York, NY: Continuum Publishing Group, 1999.

Garbarino, James. *Lost Boys: Why Our Sons Turn Violent and How We Can Save Them*. New York, NY: The Free Press, 1999.

Chapter 15
Personality Disorders

Section 1: Paranoid Personality Disorder

Books
Wouk, Herman. *The Caine Mutiny: A Novel of World War II*, 1st edition. Garden City, NY: Doubleday, 1951.

Section 4: Antisocial Personality Disorder

Books
Black, Donald W. *Bad Boys, Bad Men: Confronting Antisocial Personality Disorder*. New York, NY: Oxford University Press, 1999.

Cleckley, Harvey. *The Mask of Sanity: An Attempt to Clarify Some Issues about the So-Called Psychopathic Personality*, 5th edition. St. Louis, MO: C.V. Mosby, 1976.

Section 5: Borderline Personality Disorder

Videos/Movies
A Streetcar Named Desire (character of Blanche DuBois). Tennessee Williams. Warner Studios, 1951, 1984, 1995. Filmstrip.

Books
Cauwels, Janice M. *Imbroglio: Rising to the Challenges of Borderline Personality Disorder*. New York, NY: W.W. Norton & Company, 1992.

Kaysen, Susanna. *Girl Interrupted*. New York, NY: Random House, 1993.

Kreisman, Jerold J. *I Hate You—Don't Leave Me: Understanding the Borderline Personality*. Los Angeles, CA: Body Press, 1987.

Middlebrook, Diane Wood. *Anne Sexton: A Biography*. New York, NY: Vintage Books, 1992.

Milford, Nancy. *Zelda, A Biography*. NY: Harper & Row, 1970.

Park, Lee C., John B. Imboden, Thomas J. Park, et al. "Giftedness and Psychological Abuse in Borderline Personality Disorder: Their Relevance to Genesis and Treatment." *Journal of Personality Disorders* 6, no. 3 (Fall 1992): 226–240.

Smith, Sally Bedell. *Diana in Search of Herself*. New York, NY: Random House, 1999.

Section 6: Histrionic Personality Disorder

Books/Opera
Carmen, an opera by Georges Bizet, 1875 (character of Carmen).

Section 7: Narcissistic Personality Disorder

Books/Literature
Mitchell, Margaret. *Gone with the Wind* (Scarlett O'Hara). New York, NY: Macmillan, 1936.
Hyman, Barbara Davis. *My Mother's Keeper: A Daughter's Candid Portrait of Her Famous Mother.* New York, NY: William Morrow & Co., Inc., 1985.

Section 10: Obsessive-Compulsive Personality Disorder

Advocacy/Support Organizations
Workaholics Anonymous
World Service Organization
P.O. Box 289
Menlo Park, CA 94026-0289   510-273-9253

Books
Robinson, Bryan. *Overdoing It: How to Slow Down & Take Care of Yourself.* Deerfield Beach, FL: Health Communication, Inc., 1992.

Chapter 16
Other Conditions

Section 1: Psychological Factors Affecting Medical (Physical) Conditions

Books
Griffith, James L., and Melissa Elliott Griffith. *The Body Speaks: Therapeutic Dialogues for Mind-Body Problems.* New York, NY: Basic Books, 1994.
Ornish, Dean. *Love and Survival: The Scientific Basis for the Healing Power of Intimacy.* New York, NY: HarperCollins Publishers, 1998.

Section 2: Medication-Induced Movement Disorders

Books
Gorman, Jack. *The Essential Guide to Psychiatric Drugs.* New York, NY: St. Martin's Press, 1990.

Section 3: Other Syndromes

Books
Relational Problems: (also see Chapter 13, "Intermittent Explosive Disorder" *resources)*
Bodine, Richard J., and Donna K. Crawford. *The Handbook of Conflict Resolution Education: A*

Guide to Building Quality Programs in Schools. San Francisco, CA: Jossey-Bass Publishers, 1997.

de Waal, Frans, and Frans Lanting. *Bonobo: The Forgotten Ape*. Berkeley, CA: University of California Press, 1997.

Bereavement:

Bronte, Emily. *Wuthering Heights*. 1847.

Nuland, Sherwin B. *How We Die*. New York, NY: Alfred A. Knopf, 1994.

Piper, William E. *Adaptation to Loss Through Short-Term Group Psychotherapy*. New York, NY: Guilford Press, Inc., 1992.

Problems Related to Abuse or Neglect:

Garbarino, James, Edna Guttmann, and Janis Wilson Seeley. *The Psychologically Battered Child*. San Francisco, CA: Jossey-Bass Publishers, 1986.

Goodman, Gail S., and Bette L. Bottoms, eds. *Child Victims, Child Witnesses, Understanding and Improving Testimony*. New York, NY: Guilford Press, 1993.

Malingering:

Mann, Thomas. *Confessions of Felix Krull, Confidence Man: The Early Years*, 1st American edition. Translated from the German by Denver Lindley. New York, NY: Alfred A. Knopf, 1955.

Appendix C
Sources of Additional Information for the Layperson for Diagnoses, Medication, Psychotherapy, Referrals

Professional Organizations

Academy of Organizational and
    Occupational Psychiatry
6728 Old McLean Village Drive
McLean, VA 22101   703-556-9222

Academy of Psychosomatic Medicine
5824 North Magnolia
Chicago, IL 60660   773-784-2025

American Academy of Addiction
    Psychiatry
7301 Mission Road, Suite 252
Prairie Village, KS 66208   913-262-6161
http://www.members.aol.com/addicpsych/
private/homepage.htm

American Academy of Child and
    Adolescent Psychiatry
3615 Wisconsin Avenue, NW
Washington, DC 20016-3007
http://www.aacap.org   202-966-7300

American Academy of Clinical
    Psychiatrists
P.O. Box 3212
San Diego, CA 92163   619-298-0538
http://www.aacp.com

American Academy of Family Physicians
11100 Tomahawk Creek Parkway
Leawood, KS 66211-2672   800 274 2237
http://www.aafp.org   913-906-6000

American Academy of Pain Medicine
4700 West Lake Avenue
Glenview, IL 60025   847-375-4731

American Academy of Pediatrics
141 Northwest Point Boulevard
P.O. Box 927
Elk Grove Village, IL 60009-0927
http://www.aap.org   708-228-5005

American Academy of Psychiatry and the
    Law
One Regency Drive
P.O. Box 30
Bloomfield, CT 06002-0030
http://www.aapl.org   860-242-5450

American Academy of Psychoanalysts
47 East 19th Street, 6th Floor
New York, NY 10003   212-475-7980
E-mail: jimluce@aol.com

American Association of General
    Hospital Psychiatrists
Mount Auburn Hospital, Wyman 2
Cambridge, MA 02238   617-499-5660

American Association for Geriatric
    Psychiatry
7910 Woodmont Avenue, Suite 1050
Bethesda, MD 20814-3004
http://www.aagpgpa.org   301-654-7850

American Association for Marriage and
Family Therapy
1133 15th Street NW, Suite 300
Washington, DC 20005   202-452-0109
http://www.aamft.org

American Association on Mental
Retardation
444 North Capitol Street, NW, Suite 846
Washington, DC 20001   202-387-1968
http://www.aamr.org

American Association of Pastoral
Counselors
9504-A Lee Highway
Fairfax, VA 22031-2303   703-385-6967
http://www.aapc.org

American Association of School
Administrators
1801 North Monroe Street
Arlington, VA 22209   703-528-0700
http://www.aasa.org

American Association of Sex Educators,
Counselors, and Therapists
Howard J. Ruppel, Ed.D., Ph.D.
Executive Director
P.O. Box 238
Mount Vernon, IA 52314-0238
                        319-895-8407

American Association for Social Psychiatry
University of Louisville School of Medicine
Abell Administration Center, Room 202
323 Chestnut Street
Louisville, KY 40202-3866   502-852-6185

American Association of Suicidology
4201 Connecticut Avenue, NW, Suite 408
Washington, DC 20008   202-237-2280
http://www.suicidology.org

American Bar Association
750 North Lake Shore Drive
Chicago, IL 60611   312-988-5000

American Bar Association
Commission on Mental and Physical
Disability Law
740 15th Street, NW
Washington, DC 20005   202-662-1570
http://www.abanet.org/disability

American College of
Neuropsychopharmacology
320 Center Building
2014 Broadway
Nashville, TN 37203   615-322-2075
http://www.vanderbilt.edu/ACNP

American College of Obstetricians and
Gynecologists
409 12th Street, SW
P.O. Box 96920
Washington, DC 20090-6920
http://www.acog.com   202-638-5577

American College of Physicians
Independence Mall West
Sixth Street at Race
Philadelphia, PA 19106-1572
                        215-351-2400

American Counseling Association
5999 Stevenson Avenue
Alexandria, VA 22304   800-347-6647
http://www.counseling.org

American Group Psychotherapy
Association
25 East Twenty-First Street, Sixth Floor
New York, NY 10010   212-477-2677
http://www.agpa.org

American Music Therapy Association
8455 Colesville Road, Suite 1000
Silver Spring, MD 20910-3392
                        301-589-3300

American Neurological Association
5841 Cedar Lake Road, Suite 204
Minneapolis, MN 55416   612-545-6284

American Neuropsychiatric Association
700 Ackerman Road, Suite 550
Columbus, OH 43202   614-447-2077
E-mail: anpa@postbox.acs.ohio-state.edu

American Occupational Therapy
    Association
4720 Montgomery Lane
P.O. Box 31220
Bethesda, MD 20834-1220   301-652-2682
http://www.aota.org

American Orthopsychiatric Association
330 7th Avenue, 18th Floor
New York, NY 10001   212-564-5930

American Pain Society
4700 West Lake Avenue
Glenview, IL 60025-1485   847-375-4715

American Psychiatric Association
1400 K Street, NW
Washington, DC 20005   202-682-6000
http://www.psych.org

American Psychiatric Electrophysiology
Association
West Haven VAMAC (116A)
950 Campbell Avenue
West Haven, CT 06516
              203-932-5711, ext. 2242

American Psychiatric Nurses Association
1200 19th Street, NW, Suite 300
Washington, DC 20036   202-857-1133
http://www.apna.org

American Psychoanalytic Association
309 East 49th Street
New York, NY 10017   212-752-0450

American Psychological Association
750 First Street, NE
Washington, DC 20036-4242
http://www.apa.org   800-374-2721
                           202-336-5500

American Psychopathological Association
615 Wesley Drive, Suite 200
Charleston, SC 29407   803-852-4190

American Psychosomatic Society, Inc.
6728 Old McLean Village Drive
McLean, VA 22101   703-556-9222
http://www.psychosomatic.com/medicine

American School Counselor Association
801 North Fairfax Street, Suite 310
Alexandria, VA 22314   800-306-4722
http://www.schoolcounselor.org

American Society of Addiction Medicine
4601 North Park Avenue, Suite 101
Upper Arcade
Chevy Chase, MD 20815   301-656-3920
http://www.asam.org

American Society for Adolescent
    Psychiatry
P.O. Box 28218
Dallas, TX 75228   972-686-6166

American Society of Clinical Hypnosis
2200 East Devon Avenue, Suite 291
Des Plaines, IL 60018-4534
                           847-297-3317

American Society of Clinical
    Psychopharmacology, Inc.
P.O. Box 2257
New York, NY 10116   212-268-4260
E-mail: pross@worldnet.att.net

American Society of Internal Medicine
2011 Pennsylvania Avenue, NW
Suite 800
Washington, DC 20006-1834
http://www.asim.org   202-835-2746

American School Health Association
7263 State Route 43
P.O. Box 708
Kent, OH 44240   330-678-1601
http://www.ashaweb.org

Associated Professional Sleep Societies
1610 14th Street, NW, Suite 300
Rochester, MN 55901-2200 507-287-6006

Association for Child Psychoanalysis
P.O. Box 253
Ramsey, NJ 07446   201-825-3138

Association of Mental Health Clergy
401 Saipan Place
San Antonio, TX 78221   210-924-2940

The Beck Institute for Cognitive Therapy
      and Research
GSB Building
City Line and Belmont Avenues, Suite 700
Bala Cynwyd, PA 19004-1610
                              610-664-3020
http://www.beckinstitute.org

Canadian Psychiatric Association
441 MacLaren Street, Suite 260
Ottawa, Ontario K2P 2H3, Canada
http://cpa.medical.org   613-234-2815

Harvard Medical School
Division on Addictions
180 Longwood Avenue, Suite 330
Boston, MA 02115   617-432-0058
http://www.hms.harvard.edu/doa

International Association of Eating
      Disorders Professionals (IAEDP)
427 Whooping Loop, Suite 1819
Altamonte Springs, FL 32701
http://www.iaedp.com   800-800-8126

International Association of Psychosocial
      Rehabilitation Services
10025 Governor Warfield Parkway
Suite 301
Columbia, MD 21044-3357   410-730-7190
http://www.iapsrs.org

International Society for the Study of
      Dissociation
4700 West Lake Avenue
Glenview, IL 60025   847-375-4718

Milton H. Erickson Foundation, Inc.
3606 North 24th Street
Phoenix, AZ 85016   602-956-6196
http://www.crickson-foundation.org

National Association of Cognitive-
      Behavioral Therapists
P.O. Box 2195
Weirton, WV 26062   800-853-1135
http://www.nacbt.org

National Association of Private Psychiatric
      Health Systems
1317 F Street, NW, Suite 301
Washington, DC 20004-1105
http://www.naphs.org   202-393-6700

National Association of School
      Psychologists
4340 East-West Highway, Suite 402
Bethesda, MD 20814   301-657-0270
http://www.naspweb.org

National Association of Social Workers
750 1st Street, NE, Suite 700
Washington, DC 20002-4241
800-638-8799   202-408-8600
http://www.socialworkers.org

National Council on Problem Gambling,
      Inc.
208 G Street, NE   800-522-4700
Washington, DC 20002
http://www.ncpgambling.org/

National Education Association
1201 16th Street, NW
Washington, DC 20016   202-833-4000
http://www.nea.org
http://www.nea.org/issues/safescho/

The National PTA
330 North Wabash Avenue, Suite 2100
Chicago, IL 60611-3690   800-307-4782
http://www.pta.org/programs/sfgrdtoc.htm

Royal College of Psychiatrists
17 Belgrave Square
London SW1X 8PG, England
                          44-207-245-1231

Society of Behavioral Medicine
401 East Jefferson Street, Suite 205
Rockville, MD 20850   301-251-2790
E-mail: info@socbehmed.org

Society of Biological Psychiatry
Mayo Clinic Jacksonville
4500 San Pablo Road
Jacksonville, FL 32224   904-953-2842
http://www.sobp.org

U.S. Pharmacopeial Convention
12601 Twinbrook Parkway   800-227-8772
Rockville, MD 20852   301-881-0666

World Association for Psychosocial
    Rehabilitation
19 East 93rd Street
New York, NY 10128
                212-369-0500, ext. 2543

Federal Agencies

The Center for Mental Health Services
Emergency Services and Disaster Relief
    Branch
5600 Fishers Lane, Room 16C-26
Rockville, MD 20857   301-443-4735
http://www.samsha.gov/cmhs/cmhs.htm

The Center for Mental Health Services
Knowledge Exchange Network
P.O. Box 42490
Washington, DC 20015
800-789-CMHS (2647)   301-443-9006
http://www.mentalhealth.org

Department of Education
400 Maryland Avenue, SW
Washington, DC 20202-0498
http://www.ed.gov   800-USA-LEARN

Department of Housing and Urban
    Development
Office of Community Planning and
    Development
Office of Special Needs Assistance
    Programs
451 Seventh Street, SW, Room 7262
Washington, DC 20410   202-708-4300
http://www.hud.gov

Department of Justice
Housing and Civil Enforcement Section
Civil Rights Division
P.O. Box 65998
Washington, DC 20035-5998
                800-514-4713
http://www.usdoj.gov/crt/crt-home.html

Department of Justice
Office of Americans with Disabilities Act
Civil Rights Division
P.O. Box 66118
Washington, DC 20035   800-514-0301
http://www.usdoj.gov/crt/crt-home.html

Equal Employment Opportunity
    Commission
1801 L Street, NW
Washington, DC 20507   202-663-4900
http://www.eeoc.gov

Food and Drug Administration
Center for Drugs, Evaluation and Safety
5600 Fishers Lane, Room 12B-31
Rockville, MD 20857
                888-INFO-FDA (888-463-6332)
http://www.fda.gov/cder/consumerinfo

National Aging Information Center
Administration on Aging
330 Independence Avenue, SW
Washington, DC 2020
Eldercare Locator   800-677-1116
http://www.aoa.dhhs.gov   202-619-7501

National Center for Injury Prevention and
    Control
Mailstop K65
4770 Buford Highway, NE
Atlanta, GA 30341-3724   770-488-1506
http://www.cdc.gov/ncipc

National Criminal Justice Reference
  Service (NCJRS)
P.O. Box 6000
Rockville, MD 20849-6000   800-851-3420
http://www.ncjrs.org   301-519-5500

National Gambling Impact Study
  Commission
800 North Capitol Street, NW, #450
Washington, DC 20002
http://www.ngisc.gov

National Institute on Aging
31 Center Drive, MSC 2292
Building 31, Room 5C35
Bethesda, MD 20892-2292   301-496-9265
http://www.www.nih.gov/nia

National Institute on Aging/NIH
Alzheimer's Disease Education and
  Referral Center (ADEAR)
P.O. Box 8250
Silver Spring, MD 20907-8250
                        800-438-4380
http://www.alzheimers.org/adear

National Institute on Alcohol Abuse and
  Alcoholism/NIH
The Willco Building, Suite 400
6000 Executive Boulevard
Bethesda, MD 20892-7003   301-443-3885
http://www.niaaa.nih.gov

National Institute on Alcohol Abuse and
  Alcoholism/NIH
Office of Scientific Communication
6000 Executive Boulevard, Suite 409
Bethesda, MD 20892-7003   301-443-3860
http://www.niaaa.nih.gov

National Institute of Child Health and
  Human Development/NIH
NICHD Clearinghouse
P.O. Box 3006
Rockville, MD 20847   800-370-2943
http://www.nih.nichd.gov

National Institute on Drug Abuse/NIH
6001 Executive Boulevard, Room 5213
Bethesda, MD 20892-9561   301-443-1124
http://www.drugabuse.gov

National Institute of Mental Health
5600 Fishers Lane, Room 17-99
Rockville, MD 20857   301-443-3673
http://www.nimh.nih.gov

National Institute of Mental Health/NIH
Office of Communications and Public
  Liaison
6001 Executive Boulevard, RM 8184,
  MSC 9663
Bethesda, MD 20892-9663   301-443-4513
http://www.nimh.nih.gov

National Institute of Neurological
  Disorders and Stroke/NIH
Office of Communications and Public
  Liaison
P.O. Box 5801
Bethesda, MD 20824   301-496-5751
http://www.ninds.nih.gov

Office of Juvenile Justice and Delinquency
  Prevention (OJJDP)
810 Seventh Street, NW
Washington, DC 20531   202-307-5911
http://ojjdp.ncjrs.org

Rehabilitation Services Administration
U. S. Department of Education
330 C Street, SW, Room 3211
Washington, DC 20202-2735
                        202-205-5474
http://www.ed.gov/offices/OSERS/RSA/
rsa.html#org

Substance Abuse and Mental Health Administration's National Clearinghouse
  for Alcohol and Drug Information
11426 Rockville Pike
Rockville, MD 20852   800-729-6686
http://www.health.org

Substance Abuse and Mental Health
  Services Administration
5600 Fishers Lane
Rockville, MD 20857   301-443-4795

U.S. Department of Health and Human
    Services
200 Independence Avenue, SW
Washington, DC 20201   202-690-0257

U.S. Department of Veteran Affairs
Mental Health & Behavioral Science
    Services
810 Vermont Avenue, NW, Room 116
Washington, DC 20420   202-273-8431
E-mail: horvath.thomas@forum.va.gov

Veterans Administration
1120 Vermont Avenue, NW
Washington, DC 20421   800-827-1000
http://www.va.gov

Appendix D
Mental Health Web Site Resources for Educators, Families, and Students

Note: *Electronic Web sites about specific disorders and self-help are constantly being developed and it is not possible to provide all relevant Web sites in this book. Many Web sites will eventually link to developing sites which can be of value to teachers, counselors, students, and families. It is important to be especially alert to the origin and sponsoring individual, organization, or corporate entity for mental health Web sites. While many are well-meaning, not all represent the authority or experience of the medical and health services community and do not contain reliable, accurate information. The authors of this Primer have carefully recommended Web sites, movies, videos, and books that support educational objectives.*

E=Educators, F=Families, S=Students

Advocacy and Support

E,F   The Child Advocate—Serves the needs of children, families, and professionals while addressing medical, educational, psychiatric, legal, and legislative issues. Recommended by American Academy of Child and Adolescent Psychiatry. Also supports the "Stand for Children" program for communities.
http://www.childadvocate.net

E,F,S   Child Welfare League of America—Child Mental Health Division—An association of more than 1,300 public and private nonprofit agencies assisting abused and neglected children and families.
http://www.cwla.org/mentalh/mentalhealth.html

E,F,S   Mental Health: A Report of the Surgeon General, Executive Summary, 1999—A report asserting mental illness as a critical public health problem.
http://www.surgeongeneral.gov/library/mentalhealth/index.htm

E,F,S   Youth Violence: A Report of the Surgeon General, 2001
http://www.surgeongeneral.gov/library/youthviolence/default.htm

E,F,S   Commission for the Prevention of Youth Violence—an American Medical Association sponsored coalition of medical, nursing, and health professionals advocating a stand against violence in families and communities.
http://www.ama-assn.org/violence

Web Sites

E,F   American Medical Association Adolescent Health On-Line—A useful source about adolescents and adolescent health, aimed at health practitioners, but valuable for parents and teachers as well.
http://www.ama-assn.org/adolhlth

E,F   Combined Health Information Network (CHID)—A database containing bibliographies for education materials on health topics produced by several federal health agencies.

http://www.chid.nih.gov

F,S   Drug-Free Resource Net—A nonpartisan coalition sponsored by the communications industry to educate parents about how to communicate with their teens about drugs.
http://www.drugfreeamerica.org/parents.html

S   Go Ask Alice—Created by Columbia University's Health Education Program—a popular site for adolescents because of its confidentiality and frankness about health issues.
http://www.goaskalice.columbia.edu/index.html

E,F,S   Healthfinder—A free gateway to reliable consumer health and human services information developed by the U.S. Department of Health and Human Services.
http://www.healthfinder.gov/default.htm

S   Teen Voices Online—An online version of the magazine by, for, and about teenage and young adult women, with many articles devoted to health and social issues.
http://www.teenvoices.com

S   Think—Teenage interactive health index with articles on nutrition, mental and physical fitness, and disease.
http://www.library.thinkquest.org/25078/themind

Information Clearinghouses

E,F   Ask Eric—The U. S. Department of Education database with a broad base of subject-specific clearinghouses of research information about educational issues.
http://www.askeric.org/About

E   Center for Mental Health in Schools Clearinghouse (SMHP)—Created in 1986 at University of California to address mental health issues in schools. Features comprehensive collection of resources.
http://www.psych.ucla.edu/clearing.htm

E,F   National Clearinghouse on Child Abuse and Neglect Information—A well-established national resource of research and services for information on prevention and treatment of child abuse and neglect.
http://www.calib.com/nccanch/

E,F   National Clearinghouse on Families & Youth (NCFY)—A central resource on youth, family policy, and practice with links to other youth- and family-related Web sites.
http://www.ncfy.com

Videos/Movies

E,F,S   American Psychiatric Association Video Rental Library Catalog
http://www.psych.org/catalog/contents.html

E,F,S   American Psychological Association
http://www.apa.org/videos

E,F,S   At-Risk-Resources—Videos, posters, and curricula guides for at-risk youth.
http://www.at-risk.com

Fact Sheets and Pamphlets

E,F,S   American Academy of Child and Adolescent Psychiatry—Facts for Families and Other Resources
http://www.aacap.org/

E,F,S   American Psychiatric Association
     http://www.psych.org
     (under Public Information)
E,F,S   American Psychological Association
     http://www.apa.org/psychnet
E,F,S   National Institute of Mental Health (NIMH)
     http://www.himh.gov/publist/puborder.cfn
E,F,S   National Mental Health Association
     http://www.nmha.org/infoctr/factsheets/index.cfm
     http://www.nmha.org/infoctr/pamphlets/cfm
E,F,S   Student Counseling Virtual Pamphlet Collection—A University of Chicago virtual compilation of counseling and health pamphlets from campuses across the country.
     http://uhs.bsd.uchicago.edu/scrs/vpc/virtulets.html

Books, Journals, Newsletters

E,F,S   VOYA (Voice of Youth Advocates)—Founded in 1978, a bimonthly journal for professionals who serve teenagers from twelve to eighteen. It identifies and reviews books, Web sites, CD-ROMs, and other resources that increase understanding of teens and how to serve them. Addresses such issues as education, adolescent development, teen culture, mentoring, gender, delinquency prevention, and race. For extensive teen resources see the two following articles in VOYA:
     "You Go Girl! A Road Map to Girl Power," Katie O'Dell Madison. VOYA, June 1999, 92–96. An extensive list of books, print magazines, Web sites, organizations, and select reading list for adults who work with adolescent girls.
     "Will Boys Be Boys? Are You Sure?" Essay by Bruce Brooks, Katie O'Dell, and Patrick Jones. VOYA, June 2000, 88–92. A comprehensive listing of books, magazines, and Web sites for adolescent boys.
     http://www.voya.com/ or 1-800-462-6420
E,F   YALSA (Young Adult Library Services Association), a division of the American Library Association. This organization provides lists of juried best books for young adults and the college-bound. YALSA works with bookstores and communities to strengthen reading literacy and resources for teens. Sponsors "Teen Read Week," a nationwide program to enhance reading and use of high-quality young adult literature and media.
     http://www.ala.org/Yalsa
E,F   Youth Today—A national nonprofit newspaper for people who work with youth issues, such as juvenile detention, teen pregnancy, violence prevention, and substance abuse.
     http://www.youthtoday.org

Miscellaneous (Counseling, Statistics, Hotlines)

E,F   Community Health Status Report—An ongoing project sponsored by the U.S. Department of Health and Human Services that reports data on numerous health indicators at local levels, including major depression and recent drug use.
     http://www.communityhealth.hrsa.gov/default.htm
E,F,S   Crisis Hotlines, Toll-Free Numbers—A list for people in crisis.
     http://www.try-nova.org/tollfree.html
E,F,S   Federal Emergency Management Agency (FEMA)—The link to "Resources for Parents and Teachers" provides federal emergency plans for parents, teachers, schools, law enforcement, mental health workers, hospitals, and communities.
     http://www.fema.gov/kids/safes5.htm

Index

About the Authors

Thomas E. Allen, M.D., received his B.A. cum laude from Princeton University and his medical degree from Columbia University College of Physicians and Surgeons. He has maintained a private practice of psychiatry and psychoanalysis for over twenty-five years and is a consultant to several hospitals and health centers. He is Associate Clinical Professor of Psychiatry at the University of Maryland School of Medicine, a Fellow of the American Psychiatric Association, and a member of the American Medical Association, American Association of Private Practicing Psychiatrists, and the American Psychoanalytic Association. Dr. Allen has been President of the Medical and Chirurgical Faculty of Maryland, Baltimore County Medical Association, Maryland Psychiatric Society, Maryland Foundation for Psychiatry, Maryland Association of Private Practicing Psychiatrists, and the Baltimore-Washington Society for Psychoanalysis. He has served as a member of Maryland Congressman Benjamin Cardin's Health Advisory Committee. He is currently an Alternate Delegate from Maryland to the American Medical Association. He has published and lectured on various professional and scientific topics.

Mayer Crockin Liebman, M.D., graduated Phi Beta Kappa with a B.A. in biological sciences from Johns Hopkins University, where he was class president; he received his medical degree from New York University. He has maintained a private practice of psychiatry for over thirty years, with the additional practice of psychoanalysis for eighteen years. He has been on the faculty of Johns Hopkins University and Goucher College and is currently a member of the faculty of the University of Maryland School of Medicine. He is a Life Fellow of the American Psychiatric Association, Fellow of the International Association of Social Psychiatry, and a member of the American Medical Association, Maryland Association of Private Practicing Psychiatrists, and the American Psychoanalytic Association. Dr. Liebman has been President of the Baltimore County Medical Association, and he is currently a member of the Board of Governors of that organization and of the House of Delegates of the Maryland Medical and Chirurgical Faculty. He directed several clinical programs at Sheppard and Enoch Pratt Hospital. He has been on the staff of the National Advisory Commission on Health Facilities and a member of committees of the Surgeon General, the Health, Education, and Welfare Secretary, and the Maryland State Department of Education. He has published and lectured on numerous topics.

Lee Crandall Park, M.D., received a B.S. in zoology from Yale University and his medical degree from Johns Hopkins University School of Medicine. He has maintained a private practice for over thirty-five years, specializing in adult and adolescent psychiatry. He is Associate Professor in Psychiatry at Johns Hopkins where he is also on the Honorary Staff in the Department of Medicine. He is a Life Fellow of the American Psychiatric Association and of the American Association for the Advancement of Science, and a member of the American Medical Association, American Society for Adolescent Psychiatry, Society for Psychotherapy Research, American College of Neuropsychopharmacology, and the International Society for the Study of Personality Disorders. Dr. Park has been President of the Maryland Psychiatric Society and the Maryland Foundation for Psychiatry. He has engaged in clinical research throughout his career including studies of psychotherapy, personality disorders, and the interrelationships of psychotherapy and medication treatment, and he has published widely in journals and books. He is listed in Marquis' *Who's Who in America* and *American Men and Women of Science*.

William C. Wimmer, M.D., received his B.A. cum laude from Western Maryland College and his medical degree from the University of Maryland School of Medicine. He has been in the private practice of adult and child psychiatry for twenty years as well as the practice of psychoanalysis for fourteen years. He has also served as Chief of the Division of Child Psychiatry at Baltimore City Hospitals and Director of the Child and Adolescent Outpatient Program at Sheppard and Enoch Pratt Hospital. Dr. Wimmer is a member of the faculty of the Johns Hopkins University School of Medicine and the University of Maryland School of Medicine. He is also a supervising analyst in child analysis at the Baltimore-Washington Institute for Psychoanalysis where he currently chairs the child and adolescent committee. He is a Fellow of the American Psychiatric Association, Alpha Omega Alpha Medical Honor Fraternity, a member of the Regional Council for Child and Adolescent Psychiatry, and the American Psychoanalytic Association. Dr. Wimmer has been President of the Maryland Psychiatric Society, Maryland Regional Council for Child and Adolescent Psychiatry, and the Baltimore-Washington Society for Psychoanalysis. He has been Teacher of the Year on three occasions at Sheppard and Enoch Pratt Hospital. He has published and lectured in his areas of expertise.